STUDY GUIDE FOR

Structure & Function of the Body

FIFTEENTH EDITION

Prepared by **LINDA SWISHER, RN, EdD**

ELSEVIER

ELSEVIER

3251 Riverport Lane
St. Louis, Missouri 63043

STUDY GUIDE FOR STRUCTURE & FUNCTION OF THE BODY, FIFTEENTH EDITION

ISBN: 978-0-323-39456-7

Notices

Knowledge and best practice in this field are constantly changing. As new research and experience broaden our understanding, changes in research methods, professional practices, or medical treatment may become necessary.

Practitioners and researchers must always rely on their own experience and knowledge in evaluating and using any information, methods, compounds, or experiments described herein. In using such information or methods they should be mindful of their own safety and the safety of others, including parties for whom they have a professional responsibility.

With respect to any drug or pharmaceutical products identified, readers are advised to check the most current information provided (i) on procedures featured or (ii) by the manufacturer of each product to be administered, to verify the recommended dose or formula, the method and duration of administration, and contraindications. It is the responsibility of practitioners, relying on their own experience and knowledge of their patients, to make diagnoses, to determine dosages and the best treatment for each individual patient, and to take all appropriate safety precautions.

To the fullest extent of the law, neither the Publisher nor the authors, contributors, or editors, assume any liability for any injury and/or damage to persons or property as a matter of products liability, negligence or otherwise, or from any use or operation of any methods, products, instructions, or ideas contained in the material herein.

Content Strategist: Kellie White
Associate Content Development Specialist: Laurel Shea
Publishing Services Manager: Hemamalini Rajendrababu
Project Manager: Manchu Mohan
Cover Designer: Gopalakrishnan Venkatram

Printed in the United States of America

Last digit is the print number: 9 8 7 6 5 4 3 2

Preface

TO THE INSTRUCTOR

This Study Guide is designed to help students master basic anatomy and physiology. It works in two ways.

First, the section of the preface titled "To the Student" contains detailed information about the following topics:

- How to achieve good grades in anatomy and physiology
- How to read the textbook
- How to use the exercises in this Study Guide
- How to use visual memory as a learning tool
- How to use mnemonic devices as learning aids
- How to prepare for an examination
- How to take an examination
- How to find out why questions were missed on an examination

Second, the Study Guide itself contains features that facilitate learning. These features include the following:

1. LEARNING OBJECTIVES have been designed to break down the information to be mastered into smaller, more manageable units. The questions in the Study Guide have been developed to help the student master the learning objectives that are identified at the beginning of each chapter in the text. The Study Guide is also sequenced to correspond to key areas of each chapter. A variety of questions have been prepared to cover the material effectively and to expose the student to several different approaches to learning.
2. CROSSWORD PUZZLES, WORD FINDS, and UNSCRAMBLE THE WORDS encourage the use of new vocabulary words and emphasize the proper spelling of terms in an entertaining manner.
3. OPTIONAL APPLICATION QUESTIONS, particularly targeted for health career students, but appropriate for any student of anatomy and physiology, have been included and are based on information contained within the chapter.
4. DIAGRAMS with key features marked by numbers for identification offer tangible recall of anatomy. Students can easily check their work by comparing the diagram in the workbook with the equivalent figure in the text.
5. PAGE NUMBER REFERENCES, found in the "Answers to Chapter Exercises" section, are cross-referenced with the page in the text where the information supporting that answer is found. Additionally, questions are grouped by specific topics that correspond to sections of the text. Following each major section of the Study Guide are references to specific areas of the text that will help students who are having difficulty with a particular grouping of questions. These references will guide the students to the part of the text that they should focus their study on. These references are of great assistance to both instructor and student because remedial work is made easier and more effective when the area of weakness can be identified accurately.
6. CHECK YOUR UNDERSTANDING, found at the end of each chapter, allows students to determine how successfully they have retained the information from each section test in the chapter. By taking this final sample test of questions reviewing all areas of the chapter, students can assess their level of preparation for an evaluation by the instructor.

These features should make mastery of the material contained in the text and Study Guide a rewarding experience for both instructor and student.

TO THE STUDENT

How to Achieve Good Grades in Anatomy and Physiology

This Study Guide is designed to help you succeed in learning anatomy and physiology. Before you begin using the Study Guide, read the following suggestions. Understanding effective study techniques and having good study habits will help you become a successful student.

How to Read the Textbook

Keep up with the reading assignments. Read the textbook assignment before the instructor covers the material in a lecture. If you have failed to read the assignment beforehand, you will not grasp what the instructor is talking about in class. When you read, do the following:

1. As you finish reading a sentence, ask yourself if you understand it. If you do not, put a question mark in the margin by that sentence. If the instructor does not clear up the problem, ask him or her to clarify it for you.
2. Make sure you can perform all of the learning objectives in the text. A learning objective is a specific task that you are expected to be able to do after you have read a chapter. The objectives set specific goals and break down learning into small steps. They emphasize the key points that the author is making in the chapter.
3. Underline the text and make notes in the margin to highlight key ideas, to mark something you need to reinforce at a later time, or to indicate things that you do not understand.
4. If you come to a word you do not understand, look it up. Write the word on one side of an index card, and write the definition on the other side. Carry these cards with you, and when you have a spare minute, use them like flash cards (as you may have done when you were learning your multiplication tables). Learn how to properly pronounce and spell the word. If you do not know how to spell or pronounce a word, you will have a hard time remembering it.
5. Carefully study each diagram and illustration as you progress through the text. Many students ignore these aids, but the author included them to help you understand the material and to emphasize key areas.
6. Summarize what you read. After you finish a paragraph, try to restate the main ideas. Do this again when you finish the chapter. In your mind, identify and review the main concepts of the chapter, and then check to see if you are correct. In short, be an active reader. Do not just stare at a page or read it superficially.

Finally, approach each unit of learning with a positive mental attitude. Motivation and perseverance are prime factors in your effort to achieve successful grades. The combination of your instructor, the text, the Study Guide, and your dedicated work will lead to your success in anatomy and physiology.

How to Use the Exercises in This Study Guide

After you have read a chapter and learned all the new vocabulary it contains, begin working with the Study Guide. Read the overview of the chapter, which summarizes the main points.

Familiarize yourself with the "Topics for Review" section of the overview, which emphasizes key objectives that were outlined in the text. Complete the questions and diagrams in the Study Guide. The questions have been sequenced to follow the chapter outline and headings, and they are divided into small sections to facilitate learning. A variety of questions are offered throughout the Study Guide to help you cover the material effectively. The following are examples of exercises that have been included to assist you.

Multiple Choice Questions

Multiple choice questions will offer you options to select from, but only one answer will be correct. There are two types of multiple choice questions that you may not be familiar with that have been included in this Study Guide:

1. "None of the above" questions. These questions test your ability to recall rather than recognize the correct answer. You would select the "none of the above" answer only if all of the other possible answers for a particular question were incorrect.
2. Sequence questions. These questions test your ability to arrange a list of structures in the correct order. In this type of question, you are asked to determine the sequence of structures from the various choices given. An example of this type of question might be the following:

Which one of the following structures would be the third area through which food would pass?
a. Stomach
b. Mouth
c. Large intestine
d. Esophagus
e. Anus

The correct answer would be a.

Matching Questions

Matching questions ask you to select the correct answer from a list of options and to write the answer in the space provided.

True or False Questions

True or false questions ask you to write "T" in the answer space next to a statement if you feel the statement is correct. If you believe the statement to be incorrect, you will circle the word or words that make the statement incorrect and write the correct word or words in the answer blank.

Identify the Term That Does Not Belong

In questions that ask you to identify the term that does not belong, you are given a series of four words. Three words are given that are related to each other in structure or function. Another word is included that has no relationship to, or that has an opposing relationship to, the other three terms. You are to circle the term that does not relate to the other three terms. An example might be the following:

Iris   Cornea   Stapes   Retina

You would circle "Stapes" because all of the other terms refer to parts of the eye.

Fill-in-the-blank Questions

Fill-in-the-blank questions ask you to recall one or more missing words and insert them into the answer blanks. These questions may involve sentences or paragraphs.

Applying What You Know Questions

Application questions ask you to make judgments about a situation based on the information in the chapter. These questions may concern how you would respond to a situation or what you would suggest as a possible diagnosis when you are given a set of symptoms. These questions provide an opportunity for you to test your ability to apply the information from the chapter to practical situations.

Charts

Several charts have been included that correspond to figures in the text. Certain areas of these charts have been omitted so that you can fill them in to test your recall of these important areas.

Word Finds

The Study Guide includes word find puzzles that allow you to identify key terms in the chapter in an interesting and challenging way.

Crossword Puzzles

Vocabulary words from the "New Words" section at the end of each chapter of the text have been developed into crossword puzzles. This format encourages both recall and proper spelling. Additionally, an exercise is included that will contain scrambled words from the chapter. This, too, encourages recall and spelling in an engaging, entertaining, and challenging manner.

Labeling Exercises

Labeling exercises present diagrams with parts that are not identified. For each of these diagrams, you are to print the name of each numbered part on the corresponding numbered line. You may choose to further distinguish the structures by coloring them with a variety of colors. After you have written down the names of all the structures to be identified, check your answers. When it comes time to review before an examination, you can place a sheet of paper over the answers you have already written on the lines. This procedure will allow you to test yourself a second time without seeing the answers.

Reviewing Your Answers

After completing the exercises in the Study Guide, check your answers. If they are not correct, refer to the page listed with the answer and review it for further clarification. If you still do not understand the question or the answer, ask your instructor for further explanation.

If you have difficulty with several questions from one section, refer to the pages given at the end of the section ("If you have had difficulty with this section, review pages. ..."). After reviewing the section, try to answer the questions again. If you are still having difficulty, talk to your instructor for additional help or resources.

Check Your Understanding

This exercise, located at the end of each chapter, provides you with an opportunity to test your recall of the entire chapter. A sample test comprised of key material allows you to test your ability to retain the entire chapter after you have mastered all the individual units. It gives you a general indication of your preparation for future evaluations.

How to Use Visual Memory

Visual memory is another important learning tool. If you were asked to picture in your mind an elephant with all of its external parts labeled, you could do that easily. Visual memory is a powerful key to learning. Whenever possible, try to build a memory picture. Remember, a picture is worth a thousand words.

Visual memory works especially well with the sequencing of items such as circulatory pathways and the passageways of air and food. Students who try to learn sequencing by memorizing a list of words do poorly on examinations. If they forget one word in the sequence, then they will forget all the words after the forgotten one as well. However, if you have a strong memory picture, you will be able pick out the important features even if you have forgotten some of the lesser ones.

How to Use Mnemonic Devices

Mnemonic devices are little jingles that you memorize to help you remember things, particularly items in a sequence. If you make up your own, they will stick with you longer. Here are two examples of such devices:

1. "On Old Olympus' Towering Tops A Finn And German Viewed Some Hops." This mnemonic device is used to remember the order of the 12 pair of cranial nerves. Each word begins with the same letter as the name of one of the nerves.
2. "Roy G. Biv." A very popular mnemonic device, this one helps you to remember the order of the colors of the visible light spectrum.

How to Prepare for an Examination

Prepare for an examination far in advance. Your preparation for an examination should begin on the first day of class. Keeping up with your daily assignments makes the final preparation for an examination much easier. You should begin your final preparation at least three nights before a test. Last-minute studying usually means poor results and limited retention of the material. The following suggestions may help you improve your test results:

1. Make sure that you understand and can perform all of the learning objectives for the chapter on which you are being tested.
2. Review the appropriate questions in this Study Guide. Reviewing is something that you should do after every class and at the end of every study session. It is important to keep going over the material until you have a thorough understanding of the chapter and a rapid recall of its contents. If review becomes a daily habit, studying for the actual examination will not be difficult. Go through each question in the Study Guide and write down an answer. Do the same for the exercises in which you label each structure on a diagram. If you have already done this as part of your daily review, cover the answers with a piece of paper and quiz yourself again.
3. Check the answers that you have written down against the correct answers in the back of the Study Guide. Go back and study the areas in the text that refer to questions that you answered incorrectly and then try to answer those questions again. If you still cannot answer a question or label a structure correctly, ask your instructor for additional help.
4. As you read a chapter, ask yourself what questions you would ask if you were writing an evaluation for that unit. You will most likely ask yourself many of the questions that will show up on your examination.
5. Get a good night's sleep before the test. Staying up late and upsetting your biorhythms will only make you less efficient during the test.

How to Take an Examination

The Day of the Test

1. Get up early enough to avoid rushing. Eat appropriately. Your body needs fuel, but a heavy meal just before a test is not a good idea.
2. Keep calm. Briefly look over your notes. If you have properly prepared for the test, there will be no need for last-minute cramming.
3. Make sure that you have everything you need to take the test, such as pens, pencils, test sheets, and so forth.
4. Allow enough time to get to the examination site. Missing your bus, getting stuck in traffic, or being unable to find a parking space will not put you in a good frame of mind to do well on the examination.

During the Examination

1. Pay careful attention to the instructions for the test.
2. Note any corrections that may be given by the instructor.
3. Budget your time so that you will be able to finish the test.
4. Ask the instructor for clarification if you do not understand a question or an instruction.
5. Concentrate on your own test and do not allow yourself to be distracted by others in the room.

Hints for Taking a Multiple Choice Test

1. Read each question carefully. Pay attention to each word.
2. Eliminate obviously wrong answers and then carefully consider those that remain.
3. Go through the test once and quickly answer the questions you are sure about; then go back over the test and answer the rest of the questions.
4. Fill in the answer spaces completely. Delete any evidence of a prior answer if you make a mistake and are providing a new answer.
5. If you must guess, stick with your first hunch. Most often students will change right answers to wrong ones.
6. If you will not be penalized for guessing, do not leave any blanks.

Hints for Taking an Essay Test

1. Budget time for each question.
2. Write legibly, if the test is handwritten, and try to spell words correctly.
3. Be concise, complete, and specific. Do not be repetitious or long-winded.
4. Organize your answer in an outline. This will help you to keep your thoughts organized, and it will also help the person who is grading the test.
5. Answer each question as thoroughly as you can, but leave some room for possible additions.

Hints for Taking a Laboratory Practical Examination

Students often have a hard time with this kind of test. Visual memory is very important in this situation. To put it simply, you must be able to identify every structure you have studied. If you are unable to identify a structure, then you will be unable to answer any questions about that structure.

Examples that may appear on this sort of examination include the following:

1. Identification of a structure, organ, or feature.
2. Description of the function of a structure, organ, or feature.
3. Description of the sequence in which air flow, passage of food, elimination of urine, and so on, occurs.
4. Questions about diseases, such as "If a thyroid fails, what condition might result?" or "What disease might occur if the pancreas is not functioning properly?"

How to Find Out Why Questions Were Missed on an Examination

After the Examination

Go over your test after it has been scored to see what you missed and why you missed it. You can pick up important clues that will help you on future evaluations. Ask yourself these questions:

1. Did I miss questions because I did not read them carefully?
2. Did I miss questions because I had gaps in my knowledge?
3. Did I miss questions because I did not understand certain scientific words?
4. Did I miss questions because I did not have a good visual memory of things?

Be sure to go back and review the things you did not know. Chances are good that these topics will come up again on another examination in the future. You should have an understanding of these topics before progressing further in the course.

Your grades in other classes will also improve when you apply these study methods to other courses. Learning should be fun. With these helpful hints and this Study Guide, you should be able to achieve the grades you desire in anatomy and physiology class. Good luck!

Acknowledgments

I wish to express my appreciation to the staff of Elsevier, Inc., and especially to Kellie White and Laurel Shea. My continued admiration and thanks go to Kevin Patton and Gary Thibodeau. Your dedication to science education has given countless students an appreciation for the wonderment of the human body, inspired our future scientists, and contributed to the improvement of health care providers. Finally, this book is dedicated in memory of my beloved husband, Bill—my beautiful connection to the past—and to my children, Sam and Mandi, and my grandchildren, Billy, Maddie, and Heather—the sunshine of my life and my link to the future.

Linda Swisher, RN, EdD

Contents

CHAPTER 1

Introduction to the Body

Command of terminology is necessary for a student to be successful in any area of science. This chapter defines the terms and concepts basic to the field of anatomy and physiology. A firm foundation in these language skills will assist you with all future chapters.

The study of anatomy and physiology involves the structure and function of an organism and the relationship of its parts. It begins with a basic organization of the body into different structural levels. Beginning with the smallest level (the cell) and progressing to the largest, most complex level (the system), this chapter familiarizes you with the terminology and the levels of organization necessary to facilitate the study of the body as parts or as a whole.

It is also important to be able to identify and describe specific body areas or regions as you progress in this field. The anatomical position is used as a reference position when the body is dissected into planes, regions, or cavities. The terms defined in this chapter allow you to describe the areas efficiently and accurately.

Finally, the process of homeostasis is reviewed. This state of relative constancy in the chemical composition of body fluids is necessary for good health. In fact, the very survival of the species depends on the successful maintenance of homeostasis.

TOPICS FOR REVIEW

Before progressing to Chapter 2, you should have an understanding of the structural levels of organization; the planes, regions, and cavities of the body; the terms used to describe these areas; and the concept of homeostasis as it relates to the survival of the species.

THE SCIENTIFIC METHOD

Complete these statements regarding research.

1. A systematic approach to discovery is known as the _____.

2. A tentative explanation in research is known as the _____.

3. The testing of a hypothesis is _____.

4. A group getting a drug is the _____.

5. A group getting a substitute is the _____.

METRIC SYSTEM

True or False

If the statement is true, write "T" in the answer blank. If the statement is false, correct the statement by circling the incorrect term and writing the correct term in the answer blank.

6. _____ There is a subtle shift toward the conversion of English measurements to the metric system.

7. _____ A centimeter is 39.37 inches.

8. _____ A pound is equivalent to 454 grams.

9. _____ An inch equals approximately 2.5 cm.

10. _____ A centron is another name for a micrometer.

LEVELS OF ORGANIZATION

Match the term on the left with the proper selection on the right.

11. _____ Organism

12. _____ Cells

13. _____ Tissue

14. _____ Organ

15. _____ Systems

a. Many cells that act together to perform a common function
b. The most complex units that make up the body
c. A group of several different kinds of tissues arranged to perform a special function
d. Denotes a living thing
e. The smallest "living" units of structure and function in the body

➔ *If you had difficulty with this section, review pages 4-6.*

ANATOMICAL POSITION

Match the term on the left with the proper selection on the right.

16. _____ Body

17. _____ Arms

18. _____ Feet

19. _____ Prone

20. _____ Supine

a. At the sides
b. Face upward
c. Erect
d. Face downward
e. Forward

➔ *If you had difficulty with this section, review pages 6-7.*

ANATOMICAL DIRECTIONS—PLANES OF THE BODY

Fill in the crossword puzzle.

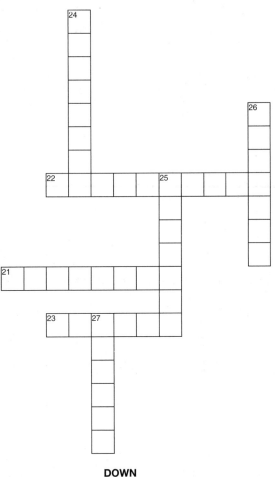

ACROSS
21. Lower or below
22. Horizontal plane
23. Toward the midline of the body

DOWN
24. Upper or above
25. Front (abdominal side)
26. Toward the side of the body
27. Farthest from the point of origin of a body point

Circle the correct answer.

28. The stomach is (*superior* or *inferior*) to the diaphragm.

29. The nose is located on the (*anterior* or *posterior*) surface of the body.

30. The lungs lie (*medial* or *lateral*) to the heart.

31. The elbow lies (*proximal* or *distal*) to the forearm.

32. The skin is (*superficial* or *deep*) to the muscles below it.

33. A midsagittal plane divides the body into (*equal* or *unequal*) parts.

34. A frontal plane divides the body into (*anterior and posterior* or *superior and inferior*) sections.

35. A transverse plane divides the body into (*right and left* or *upper and lower*) sections.

36. A coronal plane may also be referred to as a (*sagittal* or *frontal*) plane.

➡ *If you had difficulty with this section, review pages 7-9.*

BODY CAVITIES

Select the correct term from the choices given and insert the letter in the answer blank.

a. Ventral cavity
b. Dorsal cavity

37. _____ Thoracic

38. _____ Cranial

39. _____ Abdominal

40. _____ Pelvic

41. _____ Mediastinum

42. _____ Spinal

43. _____ Pleural

➔ *If you had difficulty with this section, review pages 9-10.*

BODY REGIONS

Circle the one that does not belong.

44. Axial   Head   Trunk   Extremities

45. Axillary   Cephalic   Brachial   Antecubital

46. Frontal   Orbital   Plantar   Nasal

47. Carpal   Crural   Plantar   Pedal

48. Cranial   Occipital   Tarsal   Temporal

➔ *If you had difficulty with this section, review pages 11-12.*

THE BALANCE OF BODY FUNCTIONS

Fill in the blanks.

49. _____ depends on the body's ability to maintain or restore homeostasis.

50. *Homeostasis* is the term used to describe the relative constancy of the body's _____.

51. The basic type of homeostatic control system in the body is called a _____ _____.

52. Homeostatic control mechanisms are categorized as either _____ or _____ feedback loops.

53. Negative feedback loops tend to _____ conditions.

54. Positive feedback control loops are _____.

55. Changes and functions that occur during the early years are called _____ _____.

56. Changes and functions that occur after young adulthood are called _____ _____.

➔ *If you had difficulty with this section, review pages 12-17.*

UNSCRAMBLE THE WORDS

Unscramble the circled letters and fill in the statement.

57. **L X A A I**

| ⭕ | | | | |

58. **Y Y G P H I O O S L**

| | | | | ⭕ | | ⭕ | | |

59. **N O R L A T F**

| | | ⭕ | | | | |

60. **A S R O D L**

| | ⭕ | | | |

What was Becky's favorite music?

61.

| | | | | |

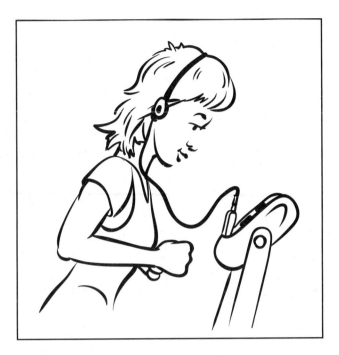

APPLYING WHAT YOU KNOW

62. Wanda has had an appendectomy. The nurse is preparing to change the dressing. She knows that the appendix is located in the right iliac inguinal region and that the distal portion extends at an angle into the hypogastric region. Place an X on the diagram where the nurse will place the dressing.

63. Mrs. Wiedeke noticed a lump in her breast. Dr. Reeder noted on her chart that a small mass was located in the left breast medial to the nipple. Place an X where Mrs. Wiedeke's lump is located.

64. Heather was injured in a bicycle accident. X-ray films revealed that she had a fracture of the right patella. A cast was applied from the distal femoral region and to the pedal region. Place an X where Heather's cast begins and another where it ends.

65. Sophia was in an accident and was transported to the hospital. She heard the paramedic mention that she had lost a great deal of blood and that her pulse was 130. She normally ran a pulse of around 84. She wondered why her pulse would not be lower as she felt her heart would try to slow down and conserve blood while attempting to clot. What would you tell her is the possible reason her pulse is so high and what feedback loop has been initiated? What emergency method could be started to stop the loss of blood until she got to the hospital? Can you suggest another example in the body where this type of loop may occur and under what conditions?

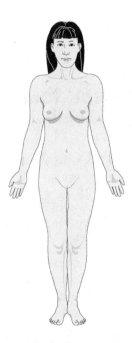

66. WORD FIND

Can you find 18 terms from this chapter in the box of letters? Words may be spelled top to bottom, bottom to top, right to left, left to right, or diagonally.

Anatomy   Posterior
Atrophy   Proximal
Homeostasis   Sagittal
Medial   Superficial
Mediastinum   Superior
Organ   System
Organization   Thoracic
Physiology   Tissue
Pleural   Ventral

```
N H L T E B W N G N M M Y X A
O O H A V U U C L W E P N G L
I M U N I T S A I D E M W A L
T E R T V C T S I C J S R T K
A O N O P T I A I W A T Y R H
Z S Q S I R L F A T N R G O W
I T W G P R O I R E T S O P F
N A A Z J E E X V E E H L H Z
A S N L M C T P I C P D O Y T
G I C A Y U O X U M N U I V P
R S M R T N U K B S A Y S V M
O R C U R O I R B S Q L Y U G
L H X E M P M E T S Y S H V S
U W L L Q D U Y Y N E E P J B
Q N Z P K D B O D C G I N J A
```

❓ DID YOU KNOW?

• Many animals produce tears, but only humans weep as a result of emotional stress.
• Men notice subtle signs of sadness in a face only 40% of the time; women pick up on them 90% of the time.

CHECK YOUR KNOWLEDGE

Multiple Choice

Select the best answer.

1. The body's continuous ability to respond to changes in the environment and to maintain relative constancy in the internal environment is called:
   a. Homeostasis
   b. Superficial
   c. Structural levels
   d. None of the above

2. The regions frequently used by health professionals to locate pain or tumors divide the abdomen into four basic areas called:
   a. Planes
   b. Cavities
   c. Pleural
   d. Quadrants

3. Which of the following organs or structures does *not* lie within the mediastinum?
   a. Aorta
   b. Liver
   c. Esophagus
   d. Trachea

4. A lengthwise plane running from front to back that divides the body into right and left sides is called:
   a. Transverse
   b. Coronal
   c. Frontal
   d. Sagittal

5. A study of the functions of living organisms and their parts is called:
   a. Physiology
   b. Chemistry
   c. Biology
   d. None of the above

6. The thoracic portion of the ventral body cavity is separated from the abdominopelvic portion by a muscle called the:
   a. Latissimus dorsi
   b. Rectus femoris
   c. Diaphragm
   d. Pectoralis

7. An organization of varying numbers and kinds of organs arranged together to perform a complex function is called a:
   a. Cell
   b. Tissue
   c. System
   d. Region

8. The plane that divides superior (upper) from inferior (lower) is known as the _____ plane.
   a. Transverse
   b. Sagittal
   c. Frontal
   d. None of the above

9. Which one of the following structures does *not* lie within the abdominal cavity?
   a. Spleen
   b. Most of the small intestine
   c. Urinary bladder
   d. Stomach

10. Which of the following is an example of an upper abdominal region?
    a. Right iliac region
    b. Left hypochondriac region
    c. Left lumbar region
    d. Hypogastric region

11. The dorsal body cavity contains components of the:
    a. Reproductive system
    b. Digestive system
    c. Respiratory system
    d. Nervous system

12. What organ is *not* found in the pelvic cavity?
    a. Bladder
    b. Stomach
    c. Rectum
    d. Colon

13. Many cells acting together to perform a common function exist at the _____ level of organization.
    a. Organ
    b. Chemical
    c. Tissue
    d. System

14. A coronal plane divides the body into _____ and _____ portions.
    a. Anterior and posterior
    b. Upper and lower
    c. Right and left
    d. Superficial and deep

15. If your reference point is "nearest the trunk of the body" rather than "farthest from the trunk of the body," where does the elbow lie in relation to the wrist?
    a. Anterior
    b. Posterior
    c. Distal
    d. Proximal

16. In the anatomical position:
    a. The dorsal body cavity is anterior to the ventral body cavity
    b. The palms face toward the back of the body
    c. The body is erect
    d. All of the above

17. The buttocks are often used as intramuscular injection sites. This region can be called:
    a. Sacral
    b. Buccal
    c. Cutaneous
    d. Gluteal

18. In the human body, the chest region:
    a. Can be referred to as the *thoracic cavity*
    b. Is a component of the ventral body cavity
    c. Contains the mediastinum
    d. All of the above

19. Which of the following is *not* a component of the axial subdivision of the body?
    a. Upper extremity
    b. Neck
    c. Trunk
    d. Head

20. A synonym for *medial* is:
    a. Toward the side
    b. In front of
    c. Midline
    d. Anterior

Matching

Select the most appropriate answer in column B for each item in column A. There is only one correct answer for each item.

Column A

21. _____ Ventral

22. _____ Skin

23. _____ Transverse

24. _____ Anatomy

25. _____ Superficial

26. _____ Pleural

27. _____ Appendicular

28. _____ Posterior

29. _____ Midsagittal

30. _____ System

Column B

a. Equal

b. Cutaneous

c. Lung

d. Extremities

e. Respiratory

f. Anterior

g. Structure

h. Surface

i. Back

j. Horizontal

DORSAL AND VENTRAL BODY CAVITIES

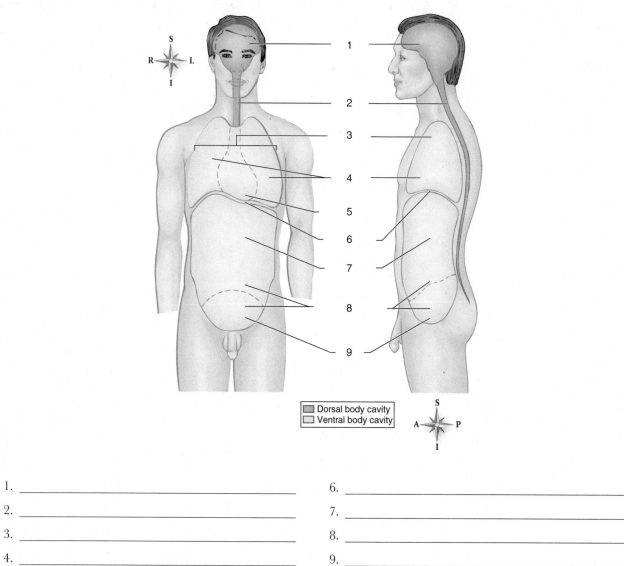

Dorsal body cavity
Ventral body cavity

1. _____
2. _____
3. _____
4. _____
5. _____

6. _____
7. _____
8. _____
9. _____

DIRECTIONS AND PLANES OF THE BODY

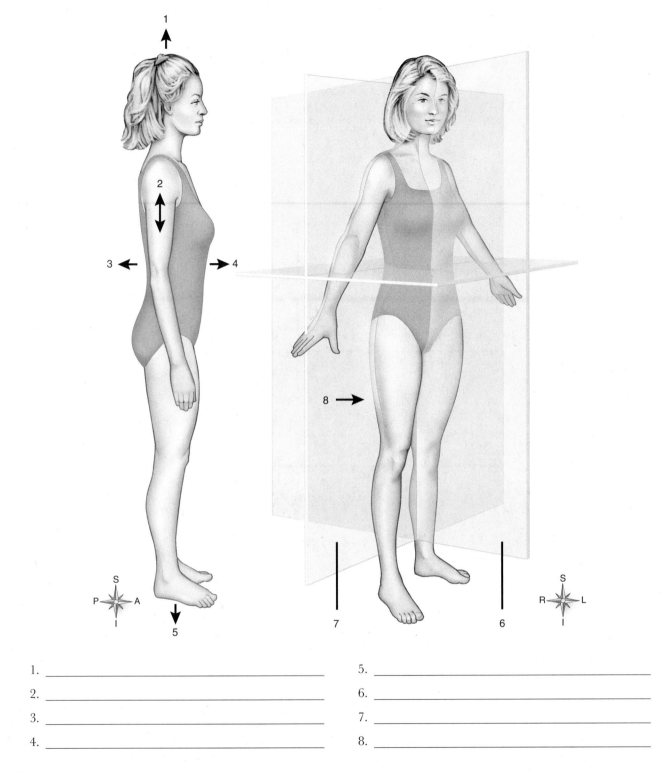

1. _____   5. _____
2. _____   6. _____
3. _____   7. _____
4. _____   8. _____

REGIONS OF THE ABDOMEN

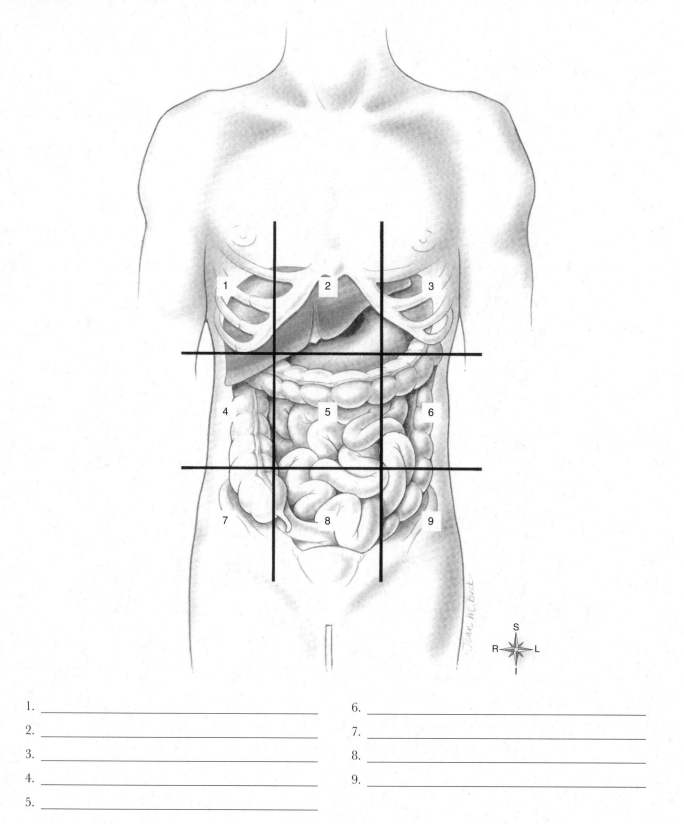

1. _____

2. _____

3. _____

4. _____

5. _____

6. _____

7. _____

8. _____

9. _____

2
Chemistry of Life

Although anatomy can be studied without knowledge of chemistry, it is hard to imagine an understanding of physiology without a basic comprehension of chemical reactions in the body. Trillions of cells make up the various levels of organization in the body. Our health and survival depend on the proper chemical maintenance in the cytoplasm of our cells.

Chemists use the terms *elements* or *compounds* to describe all of the substances (matter) in and around us. Distinguishing these two terms is the fact that an element cannot be broken down. A compound, on the other hand, is made up of two or more elements and has the ability to be broken down into the elements that form it.

Organic and inorganic compounds are equally important to us. Without organic compounds such as carbohydrates, proteins, and fats and inorganic compounds such as water, we could not sustain life.

Because we cannot see many of the chemical reactions that take place daily in our bodies, it is sometimes difficult to comprehend the principles involved in initiating them. Chemicals are responsible for directing virtually all of our bodily functions. It is, therefore, important to master the fundamental concepts of chemistry.

TOPICS FOR REVIEW

Before progressing to Chapter 3, you should have an understanding of the basic chemical reactions in the body and the fundamental concepts of biochemistry.

LEVELS OF CHEMICAL ORGANIZATION

Multiple Choice

Select the best answer.

1. Biochemistry is devoted to studying the chemical aspects of:
   a. Organic chemistry
   b. Inorganic chemistry
   c. Biology
   d. Life

2. Which of the following is *not* a subatomic particle?
   a. Proton
   b. Electron
   c. Isotope
   d. Neutron

3. Electrons move about within certain limits called:
   a. Energy levels
   b. Orbitals
   c. Chemical bonding
   d. Shells

4. The number of protons in the nucleus is an atom's:
   a. Atomic mass
   b. Atomic energy level
   c. Atomic number
   d. None of the above

5. The number of protons and neutrons combined is the atom's:
   a. Atomic mass
   b. Atomic energy level
   c. Orbit
   d. Chemical bonding

6. Which of the following is *not* one of the major elements present in the human body?
   a. Oxygen
   b. Carbon
   c. Nitrogen
   d. Iron

7. Atoms usually unite with each other to form larger chemical units called:
   a. Energy levels
   b. Mass
   c. Molecules
   d. Shells

8. Substances whose molecules have more than one element in them are called:
   a. Compounds
   b. Orbitals
   c. Elements
   d. Neutrons

True or False

If the statement is true, write "T" in the answer blank. If the statement is false, correct the statement by circling the incorrect term and writing the correct term in the answer blank.

9. _____ Matter is anything that occupies space and has mass.

10. _____ Most chemicals in the body are in the form of electrons.

11. _____ At the core of each atom is a nucleus composed of positively charged protons and uncharged neutrons.

12. _____ Orbitals are arranged into energy levels depending on their distance from the nucleus.

13. _____ The formula for a compound contains symbols for the elements in each molecule.

➡ *If you had difficulty with this section, review pages 23-24.*

CHEMICAL BONDING

Multiple Choice

Select the best answer.

14. Ionic bonds are chemical bonds formed by the:
    a. Sharing of electrons between atoms
    b. Donation of protons from one atom to another
    c. Donation of electrons from one atom to another
    d. Acceptance of protons from one atom to another

15. Molecules that form ions when dissolved in water are called:
    a. Covalent bonds
    b. Electrolytes
    c. Isotopes
    d. Ionic bonds

16. When atoms share electrons, a(n) _____ forms.
    a. Covalent bond
    b. Electrolyte
    c. Ionic bond
    d. Isotope

17. Covalent bonds:
    a. Break apart easily in water
    b. Are not easily broken
    c. Donate electrons
    d. None of the above

18. Hydrogen bonds:
    a. Do *not* form new molecules
    b. Are strong bonds
    c. Have a negative effect on body water
    d. Separate neighboring molecules, allowing them to act more effectively in other areas of the body

19. If a molecule "dissociates" in water, it:
    a. Has taken on additional ions
    b. Has eliminated ions
    c. Separates to form free ions
    d. Forms a covalent bond

➲ *If you had difficulty with this section, review pages 24-27.*

INORGANIC CHEMISTRY

Identify each term with its corresponding description or definition.

a. Aqueous solution
b. Water
c. ATP
d. Base
e. Solvent
f. pH

g. Dehydration synthesis
h. Inorganic
i. Weak acid
j. Hydrolysis
k. Strong acid
l. Reactants

20. _____ A type of compound

21. _____ Compound most essential to life

22. _____ Dissolves solutes

23. _____ Water plus common salt

24. _____ Reactants combine only after H and O atoms are removed

25. _____ Combine to form a larger product

26. _____ The reverse of dehydration synthesis

27. _____ Yields energy for muscle contraction

28. _____ Alkaline compound

29. _____ A measure of the H^+ concentration

30. _____ Easily dissociates to form H^+ ions

31. _____ Dissociates very little

➲ *If you had difficulty with this section, review pages 27-29.*

ORGANIC CHEMISTRY

Select the best answer.

a. Carbohydrate
b. Lipid
c. Proteins
d. Nucleic acid

32. _____ Monosaccharide

33. _____ Triglyceride

34. _____ DNA

35. _____ Cholesterol

36. _____ Amino acid

37. _____ Glycogen

38. _____ Sucrose

39. _____ Phospholipid

40. _____ Contains C, O, H, and N

41. _____ RNA

➔ *If you had difficulty with this section, review pages 29-33.*

CHEMISTRY OF LIFE

Fill in the crossword puzzle.

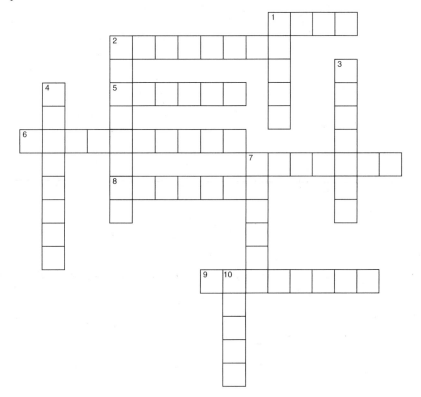

ACROSS
1. Below 7.0 on pH scale
2. Bond formed by sharing electrons
5. Occupies space and has mass
6. Reverse of dehydration synthesis
7. Substances composed of one type of atom
8. Uncharged subatomic particle
9. Subatomic particle

DOWN
1. Combine to form molecules
2. Substances whose molecules have more than one element
3. Amino acid
4. Polysaccharide
7. Chemical catalyst
10. Fat

UNSCRAMBLE THE WORDS

Unscramble the circled letters and fill in the statement.

42. **T M A T R E**

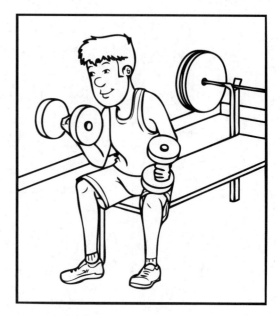

43. **S E T L M E N E**

44. **C L S M O E U E L**

45. **N A G R I O C**

46. **R L E C E T O L Y E T**

Why Bill worked out each day.

47.

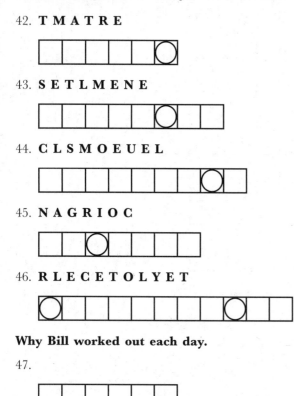

APPLYING WHAT YOU KNOW

48. Sandy just finished preparing a meal of pan-fried hamburgers for her family. While the frying pan was still hot, she poured the liquid grease into a metal container to cool. Later she noticed that the liquid oil had solidified as it cooled. Explain the chemistry of why the now room-temperature fat was solid.

49. Carol was gaining weight, yet she was eating very little. Her physician suspected hypothyroidism and suggested a test that measures radiation emitted by the thyroid when radioactive iodine is introduced into the gland. Describe what the radiologist will do to evaluate Carol's thyroid function.

50. WORD FIND

Can you find 12 terms from this chapter in the box of letters? Words may be spelled top to bottom, bottom to top, right to left, left to right, or diagonally.

Alkaline
Atomic mass
Base
Carbohydrate
Dehydration
Dissociation

Electrolyte
Molecule
Nucleic acid
Proton
Reactant
Solvent

```
E T A R D Y H O B R A C E
T B H S I H L I N A T O D
B N E H S G O U L P O T E
R Z A M S F R K U S M T H
P R O T O N A I E C I X Y
B R N U C L E I C A C I D
C A F T I A E W G G M W R
L E S N A B E C E E A E A
G Q E E T E A R U S S F T
Q R P V I B Y K I L S W I
E T Y L O R T C E L E B O
S B U O N E S P N B R B N
O P J S T D J M O L U H D
```

? DID YOU KNOW?

• After a vigorous workout, your triglycerides fall 10-20% and your HDL increases by the same percentage for 2-3 hours.
• When hydrogen burns in the air, water is formed.

CHECK YOUR KNOWLEDGE

Fill in the blanks.

1. _____ is the field of science devoted to studying the chemical aspects of life.

2. Atoms are composed of protons, electrons, and _____.

3. The farther an orbital extends from the nucleus, the _____ its energy level.

4. Substances can be classified as _____ or _____.

5. Chemical bonds form to make atoms more _____.

6. A(n) _____ is an electrically charged atom.

7. Few _____ compounds have carbon atoms in them and none has C-C or C-H bonds.

8. _____ _____ is a reaction in which water is lost from the reactants.

9. Chemists often use a(n) _____ _____ to represent a chemical reaction.

10. High levels of _____ in the blood make the blood more acidic.

11. _____ are compounds that produce an excess of H^+ ions.

12. _____ maintain pH balance by preventing sudden changes in the H^+ ion concentration.

13. _____ literally means "carbon" and "water."

14. _____ is a steroid lipid.

15. Collagen and keratin are examples of _____ proteins.

Multiple Choice

Select the best answer.

16. Two atoms that have the same atomic number but different atomic masses are _____ of the same element.
    a. Isotopes
    b. Compounds
    c. Molecules
    d. Hydrogen bonds

17. An example of an ionic bond is:
    a. NaCl
    b. Ca
    c. O
    d. P

18. The "internal sea" of the body is:
    a. Blood
    b. Aqueous solution
    c. Water
    d. Urine

19. An example of a polysaccharide is a(n):
    a. Triglyceride
    b. Enzyme
    c. Steroid
    d. Glycogen

20. ATP serves the body by:
    a. Metabolizing excess proteins in the blood
    b. Filtering harmful bacteria out of the blood
    c. Making energy available to cellular processes
    d. Serving as a catalyst for chemical reactions in the urine filtration process

CHAPTER 3
Cells

Cells are the smallest structural units of living things. Therefore, because we are living, we are made up of a mass of cells. Human cells, which vary in shape and size, can only be seen under a microscope. The three main parts of a cell are the cytoplasmic membrane, the cytoplasm, and the nucleus. As you review this chapter, you will be amazed at the resemblance of cells to the body as a whole. You will identify miniature circulatory systems, reproductive systems, digestive systems, power plants (much like muscular systems), and many other structures that will aid in your understanding of these body systems in future chapters.

Cells, just like humans, require water, food, gases, the elimination of wastes, and numerous other substances and processes in order to survive. The movement of these substances into and out of cells is accomplished by two primary methods: passive transport processes and active transport processes. In passive transport processes, no cellular energy is required to effect movement through the cell membrane. However, in active transport processes, cellular energy is required to provide movement through the cell membrane. The cellular energy required for this movement is obtained from adenosine triphosphate (ATP).

The study of cell reproduction completes the chapter's overview of cells. A basic explanation of DNA, "the hereditary molecule," provides a proper respect for the capability of the cell to transmit physical and mental traits from generation to generation. Reproduction of the cell, mitosis, is a complex process requiring several stages. These stages are outlined and diagrammed in the text to facilitate learning.

TOPICS FOR REVIEW

Before progressing to Chapter 4, you should have an understanding of the structure and function of the smallest living unit in the body—the cell. Your review should also include the methods by which substances move through the cell membrane and the stages that occur during cell reproduction.

CELLS/PARTS OF A CELL

Match the term on the left with the proper selection on the right.

Group A

1. _____ Cytoplasm

2. _____ Plasma membrane

3. _____ Cholesterol

4. _____ Nucleus

5. _____ Centrioles

  a. Component of plasma membrane
  b. Controls reproduction of the cell
  c. "Living matter"
  d. Function during cell division
  e. Surrounds and serves as a boundary for cells

Group B

6. _____ Ribosomes

7. _____ Endoplasmic reticulum

8. _____ Mitochondria

9. _____ Lysosomes

10. _____ Golgi apparatus

  a. "Power plants"
  b. "Digestive bags"
  c. "Chemical processing and packaging center"
  d. "Protein factories"
  e. "Smooth and rough"

Fill in the blanks.

11. The numerous small structures that function like organs in a cell are called _____.

12. A procedure performed prior to transplanting an organ from one individual to another is _____ _____.

13. Fine, hairlike extensions found on the exposed or free surfaces of some cells are called _____.

14. The process that uses oxygen to break down glucose and other nutrients to release energy required for cellular work is called _____ _____.

15. _____ are usually attached to rough endoplasmic reticulum and produce enzymes and other protein compounds.

16. The _____ provide energy-releasing chemical reactions that go on continuously.

17. The organelles that can digest and destroy microbes that invade the cell are called _____.

18. Mucus is an example of a product manufactured by the _____ _____.

19. These rod-shaped structures, _____, play an important role during cell division.

20. _____ _____ in the nucleus are made of proteins around which are wound segments of the long, threadlike molecules called DNA.

➲ *If you had difficulty with this section, review pages 41-48.*

MOVEMENT OF SUBSTANCES THROUGH CELL MEMBRANES

Select the best answer.

21. The energy required for active transport processes is obtained from:
    a. ATP
    b. DNA
    c. Diffusion
    d. Osmosis

22. An example of a passive transport process is:
    a. Permease system
    b. Phagocytosis
    c. Pinocytosis
    d. Diffusion

23. Movement of substances from a region of high concentration to a region of low concentration is known as:
    a. Active transport
    b. Passive transport
    c. Cellular energy
    d. Concentration gradient

24. Osmosis is the _____ of water across a selectively permeable membrane when some of the solutes cannot cross the membrane.
    a. Filtration
    b. Equilibrium
    c. Active transport
    d. Diffusion

25. _____ involves the movement of solutes across a selectively permeable membrane by the process of diffusion.
    a. Osmosis
    b. Filtration
    c. Dialysis
    d. Phagocytosis

26. An example of diffusion is:
    a. Substances scattering evenly throughout an available space
    b. An ion pump
    c. Filtration
    d. Phagocytosis

27. _____ always occurs down a hydrostatic pressure gradient.
    a. Osmosis
    b. Filtration
    c. Dialysis
    d. Facilitated diffusion

28. The uphill movement of a substance through a living cell membrane is:
    a. Osmosis
    b. Diffusion
    c. Active transport process
    d. Passive transport process

29. An example of an active transport process is:
    a. Ion pump
    b. Phagocytosis
    c. Pinocytosis
    d. All of the above

30. An example of a cell that uses phagocytosis is the:
    a. White blood cell
    b. Red blood cell
    c. Muscle cell
    d. Bone cell

31. A solution that contains a higher concentration of salt than living red blood cells would be:
    a. Hypotonic
    b. Hypertonic
    c. Isotonic
    d. Homeostatic

32. A red blood cell becomes engorged with water and will eventually lyse, releasing hemoglobin into the solution. This solution is _____ to the red blood cell.
    a. Hypotonic
    b. Hypertonic
    c. Isotonic
    d. Homeostatic

➔ *If you had difficulty with this section, review pages 48-52.*

CELL GROWTH AND REPRODUCTION

Circle the one that does not *belong.*

33. DNA	Adenine	Uracil	Thymine
34. Complementary	Guanine	Telophase	Cytosine base pairing
35. Anaphase	Specific sequence	Gene	Base pairs
36. RNA	Ribosome	Thymine	Uracil
37. Translation	Protein synthesis	mRNA	Interphase
38. Cleavage furor	Anaphase	Prophase	2 daughter cells
39. "Resting"	Prophase	Interphase	DNA replication
40. Identical	2 nuclei	Telophase	Metaphase
41. Metaphase	Prophase	Telophase	Gene

 If you had difficulty with this section, review pages 52-58.

UNSCRAMBLE THE WORDS

Unscramble the circled letters and fill in the statement.

42. **T H I R A E E N P S**

43. **E R I L C T E O N**

44. **U I I F O N S D F**

45. **O E E P A T S H L**

46. **R A N L G L E E O**

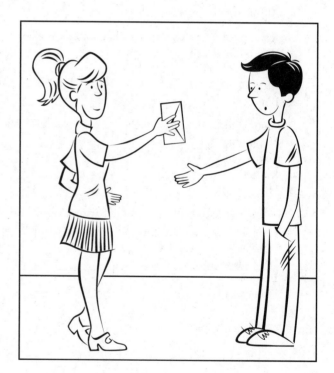

Why Susie asked Carlos to read a letter from her friend Juan.

47.

✏ APPLYING WHAT YOU KNOW

48. Mr. Fee's boat had capsized, and he was stranded on a deserted shoreline for 2 days without food or water. When he was found, it was discovered that he had swallowed a great deal of seawater. He was taken to the emergency room in a state of dehydration. In the space below, draw the appearance of Mr. Fee's red blood cells as they would appear to the laboratory technician.

49. The nurse was instructed to dissolve a pill in a small amount of liquid medication. As she dropped the capsule into the liquid, she was interrupted by the telephone. On her return to the medication cart, she found the medication completely dissolved and apparently scattered evenly throughout the liquid. This phenomenon did not surprise her since she was aware from her knowledge of cell transport that _____ had created this distribution.

50. Ms. Bence has emphysema. She has been admitted to the hospital and is receiving oxygen per nasal cannula. Emphysema destroys the tiny air sacs in the lungs. These tiny air sacs, called *alveoli*, provide what function for Ms. Bence?

51. Alice is working in the lab on a strand of DNA. The base sequence for the strand and the section that she is viewing is AGGC. What will the complementary pair be for that section of the strand?

52. WORD FIND

Can you find 15 terms from this chapter? Words may be spelled top to bottom, bottom to top, right to left, left to right, or diagonally.

```
A  P  D  I  E  V  E  W  N  P  F  E  H  Y  X
I  G  I  Z  N  S  R  L  X  S  T  W  F  Z  S
R  J  V  N  N  T  A  I  L  M  R  P  H  M  F
D  W  U  E  O  O  E  H  B  E  A  D  U  G  F
N  W  I  U  I  C  I  R  P  O  N  N  F  B  W
O  P  U  R  S  H  Y  T  P  O  S  A  W  X  K
H  X  F  O  U  R  Y  T  A  H  L  O  G  A  W
C  L  Z  N  F  O  Y  P  O  R  A  E  M  R  M
O  U  I  X  F  M  L  F  O  S  T  S  T  E  O
T  T  B  Y  I  A  B  C  O  T  I  L  E  S  D
I  V  S  O  D  T  T  M  I  T  O  S  I  S  U
M  N  A  A  I  I  L  E  N  L  N  N  N  F  R
E  O  K  K  I  D  C  Q  H  B  I  V  I  T  H
E  K  T  X  B  Z  A  E  A  L  S  A  E  C  K
S  B  Z  R  P  M  V  L  X  W  Z  A  Z  C  V
```

Chromatid	Interphase	Ribosome
Cilia	Mitochondria	Telophase
DNA	Mitosis	Translation
Diffusion	Neuron	
Filtration	Organelle	
Hypotonic	Pinocytosis	

❓ DID YOU KNOW?

- The largest single cell in the human body is the female sex cell, the ovum. The smallest single cell in the human body is the male sex cell, the sperm.
- Other than your brain cells, 50,000,000 of the cells in your body will have died and been replaced with others in the time it took you to read this sentence.

CELLS

Fill in the crossword puzzle.

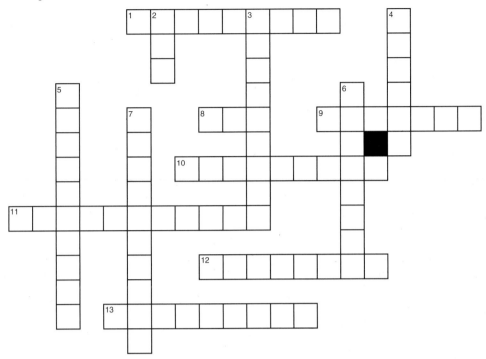

ACROSS
1. Shriveling of cell due to water withdrawal
8. Energy source for active transport
9. Reproduction process of most cells
10. Cell organ
11. Cartilage cell
12. First stage of mitosis
13. Occurs when substances scatter themselves evenly throughout an available space

DOWN
2. Ribonucleic acid (abbreviation)
3. Last stage of mitosis
4. Nerve cell
5. Literally means "center part"
6. Specialized example of diffusion
7. Having an osmotic pressure greater than that of the solution

CHECK YOUR KNOWLEDGE

Multiple Choice

Select the best answer.

1. The internal living material of cells is/are the:
   a. Cytoplasm
   b. Plasma membrane
   c. Nucleus
   d. Centrioles

2. The "protein factories" of the cell are the:
   a. Mitochondria
   b. Ribosomes
   c. Lysosomes
   d. Golgi apparatus

3. The process of enzymes using oxygen to break down glucose and other nutrients to release energy required for cellular work is:
   a. Chemical processing
   b. Cellular respiration
   c. Apoptosis
   d. Passive transport

4. Two of these rod-shaped structures exist in every cell.
   a. Centrioles
   b. Cilia
   c. Ribosomes
   d. Lysosomes

5. Adenosine triphosphate is the chemical substance that provides the energy required for:
   a. Passive transport
   b. Osmosis
   c. Active transport
   d. Dialysis

6. A solution that contains a lower concentration of salt than living red blood cells would be:
   a. Hypotonic
   b. Hypertonic
   c. Isotonic
   d. Homeostatic

7. It is the sequence of base pairs in each gene of each chromosome that determines:
   a. Anaphase
   b. Thymine
   c. Translation
   d. Heredity

8. The specific and visible stages of cell division are preceded by a period called:
   a. Anaphase
   b. Interphase
   c. Prophase
   d. Metaphase

9. Which of the following cellular structures have the ability to secrete digestive enzymes?
   a. Lysosomes
   b. Mitochondria
   c. Golgi apparatus
   d. Ribosomes

10. Red blood cells do what when placed in a hypertonic salt solution?
    a. Remain unchanged
    b. Undergo crenation
    c. Lyse
    d. None of the above

11. Which of the following statements is true of chromatin granules?
    a. They exist in the cell cytoplasm.
    b. They are made up of DNA.
    c. They form spindle fibers.
    d. All of the above

12. Filtration is a process that involves which of the following?
    a. Active transport
    b. The expenditure of energy
    c. Changes in hydrostatic pressure
    d. All of the above

13. The synthesis of proteins by ribosomes using information coded in the mRNA molecule is called:
    a. Translation
    b. Transcription
    c. Replication
    d. Crenation

14. The genetic code for a particular protein is passed from DNA to mRNA by a process known as:
    a. Transcription
    b. Translation
    c. Interphase
    d. Genome

15. All of the DNA in each cell of the body is called the:
    a. Tissue typing
    b. Genome
    c. Gene
    d. Genetic code

Matching

Select the most correct answer from column B for each statement in column A. (Only one answer is correct.)

Column A

16. _____ Endoplasmic reticulum

17. _____ Flagellum

18. _____ Chromosomes

19. _____ Passive transport

20. _____ Active transport

21. _____ Isotonic

22. _____ Transcription

23. _____ Anaphase

24. _____ Telophase

25. _____ Pinocytosis

Column B

a. Phagocytosis
b. 0.9% NaCl solution
c. Osmosis
d. Cell division complete
e. Active transport
f. Rough and smooth
g. Tail of the sperm cell
h. Cleavage furrow
i. Messenger RNA
j. DNA

CELL STRUCTURE

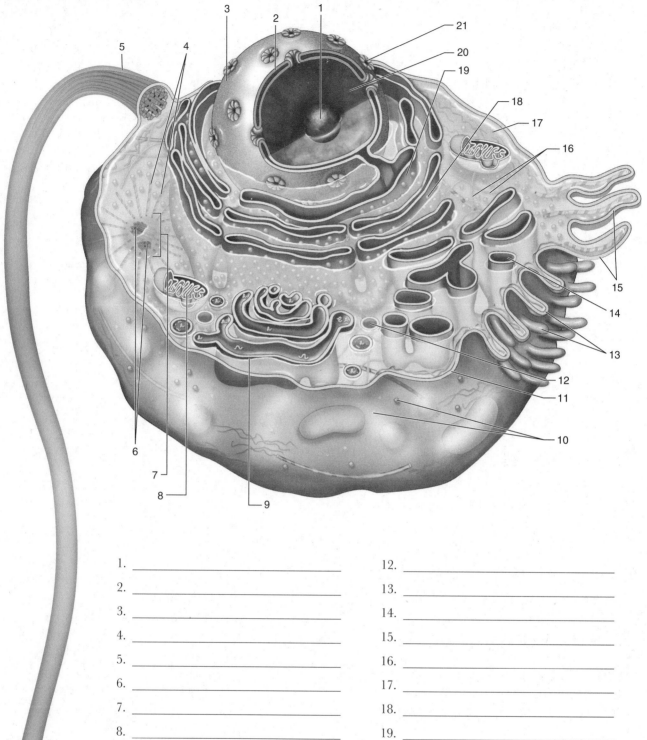

1. _____
2. _____
3. _____
4. _____
5. _____
6. _____
7. _____
8. _____
9. _____
10. _____
11. _____

12. _____
13. _____
14. _____
15. _____
16. _____
17. _____
18. _____
19. _____
20. _____
21. _____

MITOSIS

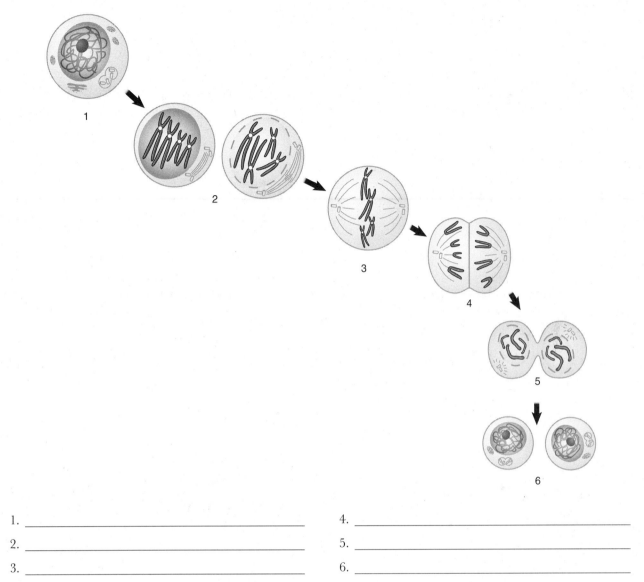

1. _____   4. _____

2. _____   5. _____

3. _____   6. _____

CHAPTER 4

Tissues

After successfully completing the study of the cell, you are ready to progress to the next level of anatomical structure: tissues. Four principal types of tissues—epithelial, connective, muscle, and nervous—perform multiple functions to assure that homeostasis is maintained. Among these functions are protection, absorption, excretion, support, insulation, conduction of impulses, movement of bones, and destruction of bacteria. This variety of functions gives us a real appreciation for the complexity of this level. A macroscopic view confirms this statement as we marvel at the fact that soft, sticky, liquid blood and sturdy compact bone are both considered tissues. As you view the various tissue slides in your text and under a microscope, you will observe the various shapes, arrangements of cells, and general characteristics of each unique type. These numerous distinctions also help to explain the varying ability of tissues to regenerate or repair after trauma, disease, or injury.

Knowledge of the characteristics and functions of tissues is necessary to complete your understanding of this structural level of organization. It will allow you to successfully bridge your knowledge between the cell and the study of body organs.

TOPICS FOR REVIEW

Before progressing to Chapter 5, you should thoroughly review the types of tissues that are present in the body. The unique characteristics of each example will allow you to easily identify them under a microscope. Additionally, it will help you understand the necessity and importance of tissues in the body.

INTRODUCTION TO TISSUES

Multiple Choice

Select the best answer.

1. A tissue is:
   a. A membrane that lines body cavities
   b. A group of similar cells that perform a unique function to help the organ do its job
   c. A thin sheet of cells embedded in a matrix
   d. The most complex organizational unit of the body

2. The four principal types of tissues include all of the following *except:*
   a. Nervous
   b. Muscle
   c. Cartilage
   d. Connective

3. Tissues differ from one another in the:
   a. Size and shape of their cells
   b. Amount and kind of material between the cells
   c. Special functions they perform
   d. All of the above

➔ *If you had difficulty with this section, review pages 67-68.*

EPITHELIAL TISSUE

Multiple Choice

Select the best answer.

4. Which of the following is *not* a function of epithelium?
   a. Secretion
   b. Protection
   c. Absorption
   d. All are functions of the membranous epithelium

5. Which of the following is *not* a structural example of epithelium?
   a. Stratified squamous
   b. Simple transitional
   c. Simple columnar
   d. Pseudostratified

6. Epithelial cells can be classified according to shape. Which of the following is *not* a characteristic shape of epithelium?
   a. Cuboidal
   b. Rectangular
   c. Squamous
   d. Columnar

7. Endocrine glands discharge their products into:
   a. Body cavities
   b. Blood
   c. Organ surfaces
   d. None of the above

8. Which statement regarding pseudostratified epithelium is false?
   a. Basement membrane lies beneath pseudostratified epithelium.
   b. Pseudo means "false."
   c. Pseudostratified epithelium is two layers thick.
   d. Pseudostratified epithelium lines the trachea.

Matching

Identify the arrangement of epithelial cells with its corresponding description.

9. _____ Single layer of cube-shaped cells

10. _____ Multiple layers of cells with flat cells at the outer surface

11. _____ Single layer of flat cells

12. _____ Single layer of tall, thin cells that compose the surface of mucous membranes

13. _____ Cilia from this tissue move mucus along the lining surface of the trachea

14. _____ Typically found in body areas subjected to stress and must be able to stretch

a. Simple squamous
b. Simple cuboidal
c. Simple columnar
d. Pseudostratified
e. Stratified squamous
f. Stratified transitional

Labeling

Label the following images and identify the principal tissue type of each. Be as specific as possible. Consult your textbook if you need assistance.

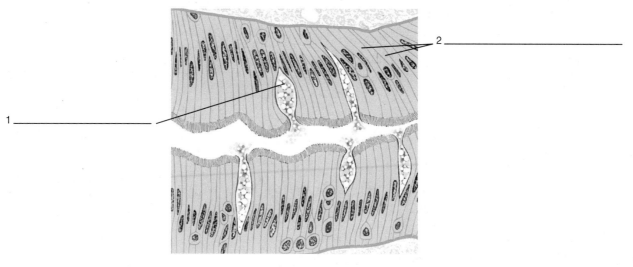

1 _____

2 _____

1. Tissue type: _____

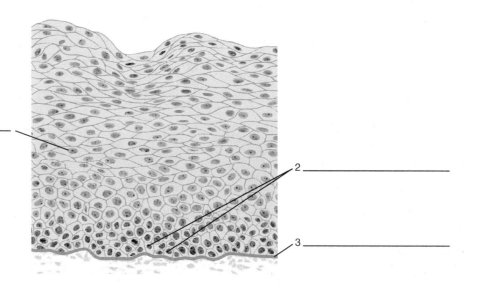

1 _____

2 _____

3 _____

2. Tissue type: _____

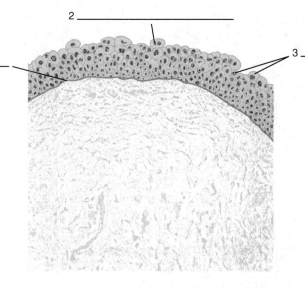

2 _____

1 _____

3 _____

3. Tissue type: _____

➔ *If you had difficulty with this section, review pages 68-72.*

CONNECTIVE TISSUE

Multiple Choice

Select the best answer.

15. Which of the following is *not* an example of connective tissue?
    a. Transitional
    b. Adipose
    c. Blood
    d. Bone

16. Adipose tissue performs which of the following functions?
    a. Insulation
    b. Protection
    c. Support
    d. All of the above

17. The basic structural unit of bone is the microscopic:
    a. Osteon
    b. Lacunae
    c. Lamellae
    d. Canaliculi

18. The term *osteon* is synonymous with:
    a. Cartilage
    b. Chondrocyte
    c. Haversian system
    d. Osteoblast

19. Dense fibrous connective tissue consists mainly of:
    a. White collagen fibers
    b. Liquid matrix
    c. Goblet cells
    d. Glands

20. Which statement is false regarding connective tissue?
    a. It is the most abundant tissue.
    b. It is widely distributed throughout the body.
    c. It exists in more varied forms than any of the other tissue types.
    d. It is voluntary.

Labeling

Label the following images and identify the principal tissue type of each.

1 _____   2

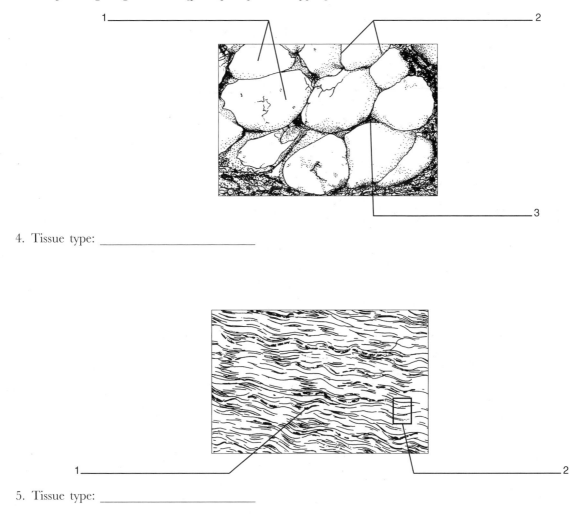

3

4. Tissue type: _____

1 _____   2

5. Tissue type: _____

1

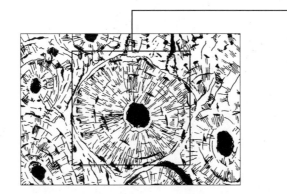

6. Tissue type: _____

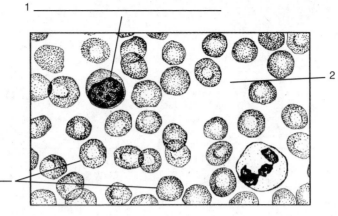

1 _____

2 _____

3 _____

7. Tissue type: _____

➜ *If you had difficulty with this section, review pages 73-76.*

MUSCLE TISSUE

Matching

Identify the type of muscle tissue with its corresponding definition.

a. Cardiac muscle
b. Skeletal muscle
c. Smooth muscle

21. _____ Cylindrical, striated, voluntary cells

22. _____ Nonstriated, involuntary, narrow fibers with only one nucleus per fiber

23. _____ Striated, branching, involuntary cells with intercalated disks

24. _____ Responsible for willed body movements

25. _____ Also called *visceral muscle*

26. _____ Found in the walls of hollow internal organs

Labeling

Label the following images and identify the principal tissue type of each.

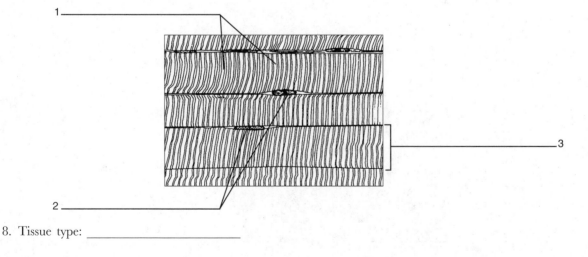

1 _____

2 _____

3 _____

8. Tissue type: _____

1 _____

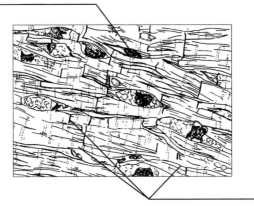

2

9. Tissue type: _____

 If you had difficulty with this section, review pages 77-78.

NERVOUS TISSUE

Matching

Match each term with its corresponding description.

a. Neuron
b. Neuroglia
c. Axon
d. Dendrite

27. _____ Supportive cells

28. _____ Cell process that transmits nerve impulses away from the cell body

29. _____ The conducting cells of the nervous system

30. _____ Cell process that carries nerve impulses toward the cell body

Labeling

Label the following image and identify the principal tissue type.

1 _____

2

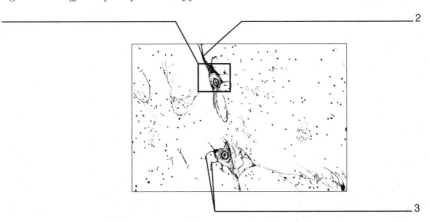

3

10. Tissue type: _____

 If you had difficulty with this section, review pages 78-79.

TISSUES

31. *Fill in the missing areas of the chart.*

Tissue	Location	Function
Epithelial		
1. Simple squamous	1a. Alveoli of lungs	1a.
	1b. Lining of blood and lymphatic vessels	1b.
2. Stratified squamous	2a.	2a. Protection
	2b.	2b. Protection
3. Simple columnar	3.	3. Protection, secretion, absorption
4.	4. Urinary bladder	4. Protection
5. Pseudostratified	5.	5. Protection
6. Simple cuboidal	6. Glands; kidney tubules	6.
Connective		
1. Areolar	1.	1. Connection
2.	2. Under skin	2. Protection, insulation
3. Dense fibrous	3. Tendons, ligaments, fascia, scar tissue	3.
4. Bone	4.	4. Support, protection
5. Cartilage	5.	5. Firm but flexible support
6. Blood	6. Blood vessels	6.
7.	7. Red bone marrow	7. Blood cell formation
Muscle		
1. Skeletal (striated voluntary)	1.	1. Movement of bones
2.	2. Wall of heart	2. Contraction of heart
3. Smooth	3.	3. Movement of substances along ducts, change in diameter of pupils and shape of lens, "gooseflesh"
Nervous		
1.	1.	1. Irritability, conduction

➡ *If you had difficulty with this section, review Tables 4-1, 4-2, and 4-3 and pages 68, 74, and 78.*

UNSCRAMBLE THE WORDS

Unscramble the circled letters and fill in the statement.

32. **E D I N E D T R**

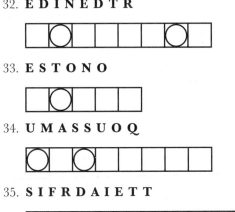

33. **E S T O N O**

34. **U M A S S U O Q**

35. **S I F R D A I E T T**

36. **L A I G**

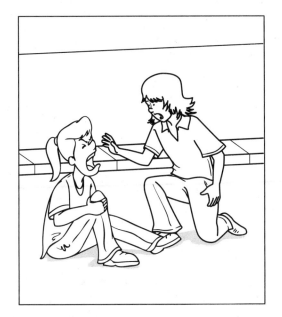

What Madison's friend gave her when she tripped and fell.

37.

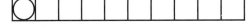

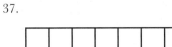

![pencil icon] **APPLYING WHAT YOU KNOW**

38. Merrily was 5′4″ and weighed 115 lbs. She appeared very healthy and fit, yet her doctor advised her that she was "overfat." What might be the explanation for this assessment?

39. Holly is a bodybuilder who is obsessed with her physique. She exercises daily and eats a very low-fat diet. A personal fitness trainer has assessed her body fat at 12%. Determine whether she is too lean or too fat. Explain the relationship between her body-fat percentage and lifestyle.

40. WORD FIND

Can you find 16 terms from this chapter? Words may be spelled top to bottom, bottom to top, right to left, left to right, or diagonally.

```
R E F K L A I L E H T I P E C D
F H Y P E R P L A S I A I V E E
F A L C I L I T Z S D V B I Y F
R E S Q S O O E G H L E F T N T
M U S C L E W I N E P I B C O R
R D W O I K M E D M T M C E I A
W B N K I A K R S A J H A N T N
C O L U M N A R R T B V R N A S
U D G Q E B C T K O J P T O R I
B W D N O I S Q I P U E I C E T
O M B X I O N F J O X S L I N I
I R H R D Z A H K I T O A R E O
D O H U A P Y L R E N P G B G N
A G E H W A F T H T K I E T E A
L S D F B Y A P T I N D H D R L
P R H Q I M J W R C U A X O N C
```

Adipose	Epithelial	Muscle
Axon	Fascia	Pseudostratified
Cartilage	Hematopoietic	Regeneration
Columnar	Hyperplasia	Transitional
Connective	Keloid	
Cuboidal	Matrix	

❓ DID YOU KNOW?

- As many as 500,000 Americans die from cancer each year. That's more than all the lives lost in the past 100 years by the U.S. military forces.
- Half of all cancers are diagnosed in people under the age of 67.
- Your smell or body odor is unique to you unless you have a twin. Even babies recognize the scent on their mother.

TISSUES

Fill in the crossword puzzle.

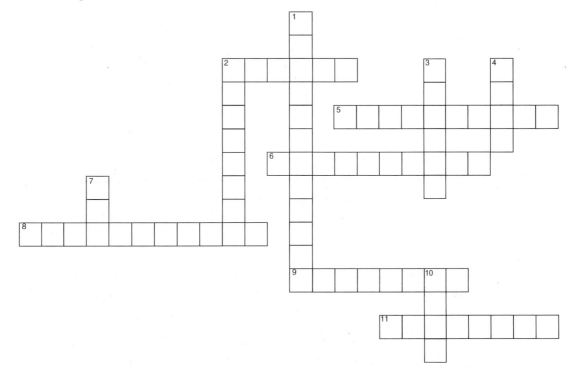

ACROSS
2. Visceral muscle tissue
5. Many layers of epithelial cells
6. Most abundant tissue in body
8. Person who studies tissues
9. Voluntary
11. Glands that release substances through ducts

DOWN
1. Cartilage cells
2. Flat, scalelike epithelial cells
3. Extracellular substance of a tissue
4. Supporting cells of nervous system
7. Adipose
10. Carries nerve impulses away from the cell body

CHECK YOUR KNOWLEDGE
Labeling

Label the following images and identify the principal tissue type of each. Be as specific as possible. Consult your textbook if you need assistance.

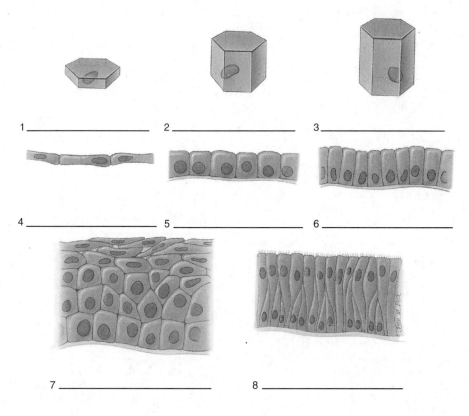

1 _____   2 _____   3 _____

4 _____   5 _____   6 _____

7 _____   8 _____

Multiple Choice

Select the best answer.

9. Which of the following is *not* an example of connective tissue?
   a. Striated
   b. Areolar
   c. Reticular
   d. Hematopoietic

10. Which of the following is the most abundant and widely distributed type of body tissue?
    a. Epithelial
    b. Connective
    c. Muscle
    d. Nerve

11. Simple, squamous epithelial tissue is made up of which of the following?
    a. A single layer of long, narrow cells
    b. Several layers of long, narrow cells
    c. A single layer of very thin and irregularly shaped cells
    d. Several layers of flat, scale-like cells

12. Which of the following groupings is correct when describing one of the muscle cell types?
    a. Visceral, striated, involuntary
    b. Skeletal, smooth, voluntary
    c. Cardiac, smooth, involuntary
    d. Skeletal, striated, voluntary

13. Cartilage cells are called:
    a. Fibrocartilage
    b. Chondrocytes
    c. Hyaline
    d. Osteocytes

Fill in the blanks.

14. _____ connective tissue is the "glue" that helps keep the organs of the body together.

15. Mucus-producing cells that appear in simple columnar epithelium are known as _____ cells.

16. The extracellular substance of a tissue is the _____.

17. The thick dark bands in cardiac muscle tissue are called _____ _____.

18. A protein that gives tissue flexible strength is _____.

19. Fascia is made up primarily of _____ tissue.

20. Another name for spongy bone is _____.

CHAPTER 5
Organ Systems

A smooth-running automobile is the result of many systems harmoniously working together. The engine, the fuel system, the exhaust system, the brake system, and the cooling system are but a few of the many complex structural units that the automobile as a whole relies on to keep it functioning smoothly. So it is with the human body. We, too, depend on the successful performance of many individual systems working together to create and maintain a healthy human being.

When you have completed your review of the 11 major organ systems and the organs that make up these systems, you will find your understanding of the performance of the body as a whole much more meaningful.

TOPICS FOR REVIEW

Before progressing to Chapter 6, you should have an understanding of the 11 major organ systems and be able to identify the organs that are included in each system.

ORGAN SYSTEMS OF THE BODY

Match the term on the left with the proper selection on the right.

Group A

1. _____ Integumentary
2. _____ Skeletal
3. _____ Muscular
4. _____ Nervous
5. _____ Endocrine

   a. Hair
   b. Spinal cord
   c. Hormones
   d. Tendons
   e. Joints

Group B

6. _____ Circulatory
7. _____ Lymphatic
8. _____ Urinary
9. _____ Digestive
10. _____ Respiratory
11. _____ Reproductive

   a. Esophagus
   b. Ureters
   c. Larynx
   d. Genitalia
   e. Spleen
   f. Capillaries

*Circle the one that does **not** belong.*

12. Pharynx   Trachea   Mouth   Alveoli
13. Uterus   Rectum   Gonads   Prostate
14. Veins   Arteries   Heart   Pancreas
15. Pineal   Bladder   Ureters   Urethra
16. Cardiac   Smooth   Joints   Voluntary
17. Pituitary   Brain   Spinal cord Nerves
18. Cartilage   Joints   Ligaments   Tendons
19. Hormones   Pituitary   Pancreas   Appendix
20. Thymus   Nails   Hair   Oil glands
21. Esophagus   Pharynx   Mouth   Trachea
22. Thymus   Spleen   Tonsils   Liver

Fill in the missing areas.

System	Organs	Function
23. Integumentary	Skin, nails, hair, sense receptors, sweat glands, oil glands	
24. Skeletal		Support, movement, storage of minerals, blood formation
25. Muscular	Muscles	
26.	Brain, spinal cord, nerves	Communication, integration, control, recognition of sensory stimuli
27. Endocrine		Secretion of hormones, communication, integration, control
28. Circulatory	Heart, blood vessels	
29. Lymphatic		Transportation, immunity
30.	Kidneys, ureters, bladder, urethra	Elimination of wastes, electrolyte balance, acid-base balance, water balance
31. Digestive		Digestion of food, absorption of nutrients
32.	Nose, pharynx, larynx, trachea, bronchi, lungs	Exchange of gases in the lungs, regulation of acid-base balance
33. Reproductive		Survival of species, production of sex cells, fertilization, development, birth, nourishment of offspring, production of hormones

➡ *If you had difficulty with this section, review pages 85-95 and the chapter summary on pages 95-96.*

UNSCRAMBLE THE WORDS

Unscramble the circled letters and fill in the statement.

34. **R T A H E**

    □ □ □ ◯ □

35. **I E P L N A**

    □ □ ◯ ◯ □ □

36. **E E N V R**

    □ □ □ ◯ □

37. **S U H E S O P G A**

    □ ◯ ◯ □ □ □ □ ◯ □

The more thoroughly you review this chapter, the less _____ you will be during your test.

38.

    □ □ □ □ □ □ □

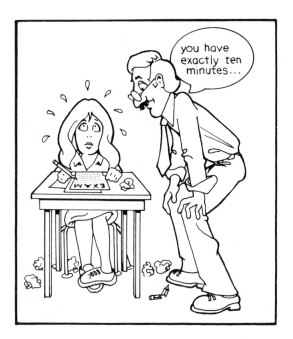

APPLYING WHAT YOU KNOW

39. Myrna was 15 years old and had not yet started menstruating. Her family physician decided to consult two other physicians, each of whom specialized in a different system. Specialists in the areas of _____ and _____ were consulted.

40. Sally's homework assignment was to explain why the nervous and endocrine systems are sometimes thought of as the "neuroendocrine system." How would you answer this assignment and support it with examples?

41. WORD FIND

Can you find 11 organ systems? Words may be spelled top to bottom, bottom to top, right to left, left to right, or diagonally.

```
Y R A T N E M U G E T N I R F
H N E R V O U S K I R J M G T
L Y M P H A T I C I S Y Y U I
B N X Y R O T A L U C R I C W
P E L R E O M J M S O M M P S
C C W M A N D L A T E L E K S
R R K E M L I U A A V V U K N
D K X P D J U R C J I R Q E M
C D B V C V I C C T T K W C X
X R Q Q D P H C S O I X P A Z
M F M U S Y D E V U D V Y K E
U E S E C Z G T Q D M N E K O
P Y R A N I R U C T C N E W H
N H T N D E P S I X A Q O I E
```

Circulatory   Lymphatic   Respiratory
Digestive   Muscular   Skeletal
Endocrine   Nervous   Urinary
Integumentary   Reproductive

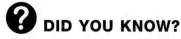 **DID YOU KNOW?**

- Muscles comprise 40 percent of your body weight. Your skeleton, however, accounts for only 18 percent of your body weight.
- Every person has a unique tongue print.

ORGAN SYSTEMS

Fill in the crossword puzzle.

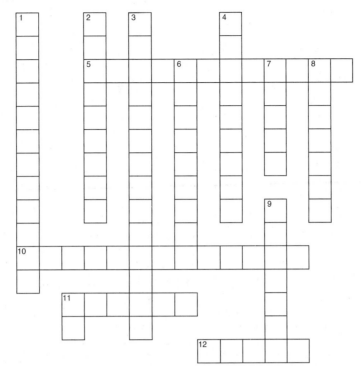

ACROSS
5. Specialized signal of nervous system (two words)
10. Skin
11. Testes and ovaries
12. Undigested residue of digestion

DOWN
1. Inflammation of the appendix
2. Vulva, penis, and scrotum
3. Heart and blood vessels
4. Subdivision of circulatory system
6. System of hormones
7. Waste product of kidneys
8. Agent that causes change in the activity of a structure
9. Chemical secretion of endocrine system
11. Gastrointestinal tract (abbreviation)

CHECK YOUR KNOWLEDGE

Multiple Choice

Select the best answer.

1. Hormones belong to which body system?
   a. Nervous
   b. Integumentary
   c. Muscular
   d. Endocrine

2. The spleen belongs to which body system?
   a. Circulatory
   b. Urinary
   c. Lymphatic
   d. Digestive

3. Which of the following is *not* an accessory organ of the female reproductive system?
   a. Fallopian tubes
   b. Mammary glands
   c. Gonads
   d. Vagina

4. The largest and most complex structural units are:
   a. Cells
   b. Organ systems
   c. Tissues
   d. Nerve impulses

5. An important function of the skeletal system is:
   a. Recognition of sensory stimuli
   b. Regulation of acid-base balance in the body
   c. Elimination of wastes in the body
   d. Formation of blood cells

6. Accessory structures of the integumentary system include all of the following *except:*
   a. Hormones
   b. Sweat glands
   c. Oil-producing glands
   d. Nails

7. Which of the following is *not* a primary organ of the digestive system?
   a. Mouth
   b. Liver
   c. Esophagus
   d. Rectum

8. One of the primary functions of the nervous system is:
   a. Communication among body functions
   b. Protection
   c. Regulation of acid-base balance
   d. Secretion of hormones

9. Which of the following is *not* an endocrine gland?
   a. Vas deferens
   b. Thymus
   c. Pineal
   d. Pituitary

10. A structure made up of two or more kinds of tissues organized to perform a more complex function than any tissue alone is a(n):
    a. System
    b. Tissue
    c. Organ
    d. Cell

Matching

Select the most correct answer from column B for each statement in column A. (Only one answer is correct.)

Column A

11. _____ Oil glands

12. _____ Blood vessels

13. _____ Tonsils

14. _____ Vas deferens

15. _____ Ureters

16. _____ Appendix

17. _____ Vulva

18. _____ Larynx

19. _____ Brain

20. _____ Thyroid

Column B

a. Endocrine

b. Urinary

c. Integumentary

d. Circulatory

e. Respiratory

f. Digestive

g. Male reproductive

h. Lymphatic

i. Female reproductive

j. Nervous

CHAPTER 6

Skin and Membranes

More of our time, attention, and money are spent on this system than any other one. Every time we look into a mirror, we become aware of the integumentary system as we observe our skin, hair, nails, and the appendages that give luster and comfort to this system. The discussion of the skin begins with the structure and function of the two primary layers—the epidermis and the dermis. It continues with an examination of the appendages of the skin, which include the hair, receptors, nails, sebaceous glands, and sudoriferous glands. Your study of skin concludes with a review of one of the most serious and frequent threats to the skin—burn injury. An understanding of the integumentary system provides you with an appreciation of the danger that severe burns pose to this system and the body.

Membranes are thin, sheetlike structures that cover, protect, anchor, or lubricate body surfaces, cavities, and organs. The two major categories of membranes are epithelial and connective. Each type is located in specific areas of the body and is vulnerable to specific disease conditions. Knowledge of the location and function of these membranes prepares you for the study of their relationship to other systems and to the body as a whole.

TOPICS FOR REVIEW

Before progressing to Chapter 7, you should have an understanding of the skin and its appendages. You should be aware of the various types of skin cancers and the ABCDE rule of self-examination of moles for early detection of skin cancer. Your review should also include the classification of burns and the method used to estimate the percentage of body surface area affected by burn injury. Knowledge of the types of body membranes, their location, and their function is also necessary as you complete your study of this chapter.

CLASSIFICATION OF BODY MEMBRANES

Select the best answer.

a. Cutaneous
b. Serous
c. Mucous
d. Synovial

1. _____ Pleura

2. _____ Lines joint spaces

3. _____ Respiratory tract

4. _____ Skin

5. _____ Peritoneum

6. _____ Contains no epithelium

7. _____ Urinary tract

8. _____ Lines body surfaces that open directly to the exterior

➡ *If you had difficulty with this section, review pages 103-106.*

THE SKIN

Match the term on the left with the proper selection on the right.

Group A

9. _____ Integumentary system

10. _____ Epidermis

11. _____ Dermis

12. _____ Subcutaneous

13. _____ Cutaneous membrane

a. Outermost layer of skin
b. Deeper of the two layers of skin
c. Hypodermis
d. The skin is the primary organ
e. Composed of dermis and epidermis

Group B

14. _____ Keratin

15. _____ Melanin

16. _____ Stratum corneum

17. _____ Dermal papillae

18. _____ Cyanosis

a. Protective protein
b. Blue-gray color of skin resulting from a decrease in oxygen
c. Parallel rows of tiny bumps
d. Brown pigment
e. Outer layer of epidermis

Select the correct term from the choices given and write the letter in the answer blank.

a. Epidermis
b. Dermis

19. _____ Tightly packed epithelial cells

20. _____ Nerves

21. _____ Fingerprints

22. _____ Melanin

23. _____ Keratin

24. _____ Connective tissue

25. _____ Follicle

26. _____ Sebaceous gland (oil gland)

27. _____ Sweat gland

28. _____ More cellular than other layer

➡ *If you had difficulty with this section, review pages 106-108.*

Fill in the blanks.

29. The most important functions of the skin are _____, _____ _____, _____ _____ _____, _____, and _____ _____ _____.

30. _____ prevents the sun's ultraviolet rays from penetrating the interior of the body.

31. The hair of a newborn infant is called _____.

32. Hair growth begins from a small cap-shaped cluster of cells called the _____ _____.

33. The nail body nearest the root has a crescent-shaped white area known as the _____, or "little moon."

34. The _____ _____ muscles produce "goose pimples."

35. Meissner's corpuscle is generally located rather close to the skin's surface and is capable of detecting sensations of _____ _____.

36. The most numerous, important, and widespread sweat glands in the body are the _____ sweat glands.

37. The _____ sweat glands are found primarily in the axilla and in the pigmented skin areas around the genitals.

38. _____ has been described as "nature's skin cream."

SKIN CANCER

Select the best answer.

39. HHV8 causes:
    a. Squamous cell carcinoma
    b. Basal cell carcinoma
    c. Melanoma
    d. Kaposi's sarcoma

40. The most serious form of skin cancer is:
    a. Squamous cell
    b. Basal cell
    c. Melanoma
    d. An epidermal mole

41. Squamous cell carcinoma is a:
    a. Slowly growing carcinoma of the epidermis
    b. Fast growing carcinoma of the epidermis
    c. Slowly growing carcinoma of the dermis
    d. Fast growing carcinoma of the dermis

42. Basal cell carcinoma:
    a. Is a rare type of skin cancer
    b. Is a common type of skin cancer
    c. Is a type of skin cancer that usually appears on the extremities
    d. Metastasizes rapidly

43. The most important factor in causing common skin cancers is:
    a. Genetic predisposition
    b. Lack of vitamin D
    c. Exposure to the sun's ultraviolet (UV) radiation
    d. Dry, scaly skin

Circle the correct answer.

44. A first-degree burn (*will* or *will not*) blister.

45. A second-degree burn (*will* or *will not*) scar.

46. A third-degree burn (*will* or *will not*) have pain immediately.

47. According to the "rule of nines," the body is divided into (*9* or *11*) areas of 9%.

48. Destruction of the subcutaneous layer occurs in (*second* or *third*)-degree burns.

➡ *If you had difficulty with this section, review pages 107-115.*

UNSCRAMBLE THE WORDS

Unscramble the circled letters and fill in the statement.

49. **P I D E E M I R S**

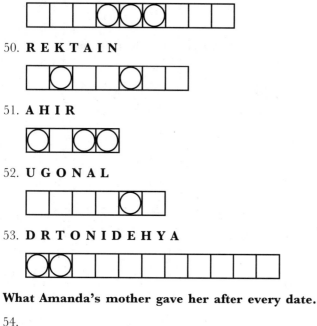

50. **R E K T A I N**

51. **A H I R**

52. **U G O N A L**

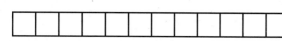

53. **D R T O N I D E H Y A**

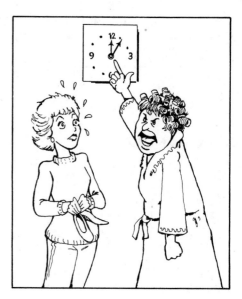

What Amanda's mother gave her after every date.

54.

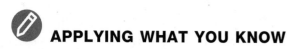

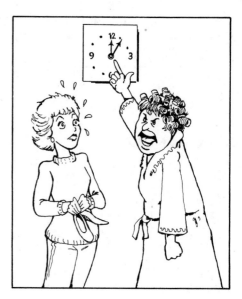

APPLYING WHAT YOU KNOW

55. Mr. Ziven was admitted to the hospital with second- and third-degree burns. Both arms, anterior trunk, right anterior leg, and genital region were affected by the burns. The doctor quickly estimated that _____% of Mr. Ziven's body had been burned.

56. Mrs. Shearer complained to her doctor that she had severe pain in her chest and feared that she was having a heart attack. An electrocardiogram revealed nothing unusual, but Mrs. Shearer insisted that every time she took a breath she experienced pain. What might be the cause of Mrs. Shearer's pain?

57. Brian was admitted to the hospital with second- and third-degree burns that covered 50% of his body. He was placed in isolation, so when Jenny went to visit him, she was required to wear a hospital gown and mask. Why was Brian placed in isolation? Why was Jenny required to wear special attire?

58. WORD FIND

Can you find the 15 terms from this chapter in the box of letters? Words may be spelled top to bottom, bottom to top, right to left, left to right, or diagonally.

```
S  U  D  O  R  I  F  E  R  O  U  S  V  K  R
E  J  U  Q  U  E  S  T  E  C  N  O  H  Y  U
I  S  J  L  M  E  L  A  N  O  C  Y  T  E  H
R  I  M  U  E  N  O  T  I  R  E  P  H  S  B
O  M  K  N  V  A  S  T  R  L  A  N  U  G  O
T  R  G  U  F  G  A  U  C  E  G  O  V  W  D
A  E  A  L  P  R  D  I  O  N  T  F  D  R  N
L  D  V  A  D  M  L  C  P  D  H  S  L  Z  F
I  I  N  Y  N  L  R  L  A  M  E  N  I  R  E
P  P  H  Q  O  N  E  U  X  R  R  F  E  L  G
E  E  Z  F  J  U  M  Y  O  U  U  O  C  C  B
D  Z  P  E  R  J  Y  U  V  F  C  I  I  E  O
G  J  S  I  W  J  S  K  C  D  T  N  O  Z  C
C  O  S  M  Z  M  F  I  B  U  G  U  X  O  J
X  Y  P  M  E  I  W  E  C  V  S  U  G  B  I
```

Apocrine	Epidermis	Mucus
Blister	Follicle	Peritoneum
Cuticle	Lanugo	Pleurisy
Dehydration	Lunula	Serous
Depilatories	Melanocyte	Sudoriferous

❓ DID YOU KNOW?

- Because the dead cells of the epidermis are constantly being worn and washed away, we get a new outer skin layer every 27 days.
- In your lifetime, you will shed 40 pounds of skin.
- *Blype* is the skin that peels off after a bad sunburn.
- Your fingernails will grow 84 feet in your lifetime.

SKIN/BODY MEMBRANES

Fill in the crossword puzzle.

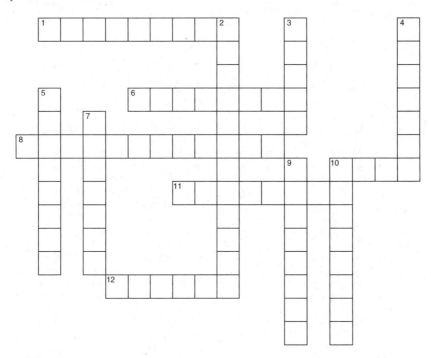

ACROSS
1. Oil gland
6. Blue-gray color of skin due to decreased oxygen
8. "Goose pimples" (two words)
10. Cutaneous
11. Inflammation of the serous membrane that lines the chest and covers the lungs
12. Deeper of the two primary skin layers

DOWN
2. Sweat gland
3. Cushionlike sac found between moving body parts
4. Brown pigment
5. Forms the lining of serous body cavities
7. Tough waterproof substance that protects body from excess fluid loss
9. Covers the surface of organs found in serous body cavities
10. Membrane that lines joint spaces

CHECK YOUR KNOWLEDGE

Multiple Choice

Select the best answer.

1. The type of membrane that lines body cavities that open directly to the exterior is known as:
   a. Mucous
   b. Serous
   c. Cutaneous
   d. Synovial

2. The dermis is the:
   a. Outermost layer of skin
   b. Deeper of the two layers of skin
   c. Layer of skin where keratin is located
   d. Layer of skin where melanin is located

3. The upper region of the dermis is characterized by parallel rows of tiny bumps known as:
   a. Dermal papillae
   b. Stratum corneum
   c. Stratum germinativum
   d. Blisters

4. One of nature's most unique proteins provides cells with an abrasion-resistant and protective quality. It is known as:
   a. Stratum germinativum
   b. Dermal papilla
   c. Melanin
   d. Keratin

5. If blood oxygen levels decrease or if actual blood flow is reduced dramatically, a condition known as _____ occurs.
   a. Lanugo
   b. Cyanosis
   c. Lunula
   d. Goosebumps

6. The hair papilla is nourished by the:
   a. Shaft
   b. Arrector pili
   c. Meissner corpuscle
   d. Dermal blood vessel

7. A Pacini corpuscle detects sensations of:
   a. Heat
   b. Pressure deep in the dermis
   c. Low-frequency vibration
   d. Pain

8. The "little moon" of your nail is the:
   a. Cuticle
   b. Lunula
   c. Nail body
   d. Nail bed

9. Which sweat glands are the most numerous and are, with few exceptions, distributed over the total body surface?
   a. Apocrine
   b. Sebaceous
   c. Eccrine
   d. None of the above

10. Because it prevents drying and cracking, this secretion is sometimes referred to as "nature's skin cream." It is more commonly called:
    a. Lanugo
    b. Sebum
    c. Perspiration
    d. Keratin

Matching

Select the most correct answer from column B for each statement in column A. (Only one answer is correct.)

Column A

11. _____ Cutaneous membrane

12. _____ Visceral pleura

13. _____ Pleurisy

14. _____ Mucous membrane

15. _____ Synovial membrane

16. _____ Subcutaneous tissue

17. _____ Lanugo

18. _____ Arrector pili

19. _____ Meissner's corpuscle

20. _____ Apocrine

Column B

a. Light touch
b. Inflammation of pleura
c. Skin
d. Serous membrane
e. Goosebumps
f. Sweat gland
g. Lines respiratory tract
h. Hypodermis
i. Bursae
j. Soft, newborn hair

Completion

Complete the phrases below with the following terms.

a. Basal cell
b. Chest cavity
c. Sudoriferous
d. Third-degree
e. First-degree
f. Joints
g. Second-degree
h. Melanoma
i. Partial-thickness burns
j. Axilla

21. The most common type of skin cancer is _____.

22. The most serious form of skin cancer is _____.

23. Pleurisy is a painful condition of the serous membrane that lines the _____.

24. The synovial membranes line spaces between _____.

25. First- and second-degree burns are called _____.

26. A typical sunburn may be classified as a(n) _____ burn.

27. Blisters are typical of a(n) _____ burn.

28. A burn that is insensitive to pain immediately after injury because of the destruction of nerve endings is most likely a(n) _____ burn.

29. Apocrine glands are found primarily in the _____.

30. The most numerous of the skin glands are the _____.

LONGITUDINAL SECTION OF THE SKIN

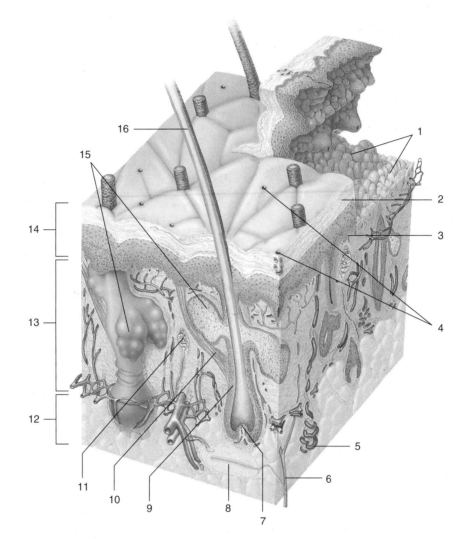

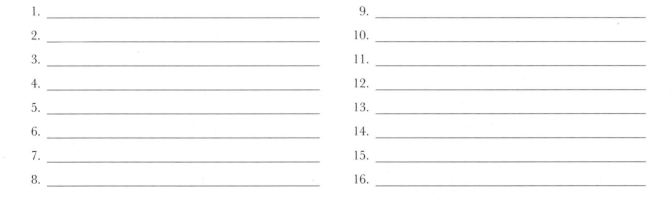

1. _____	9. _____
2. _____	10. _____
3. _____	11. _____
4. _____	12. _____
5. _____	13. _____
6. _____	14. _____
7. _____	15. _____
8. _____	16. _____

"RULE OF NINES" FOR ESTIMATING SKIN SURFACE BURNED

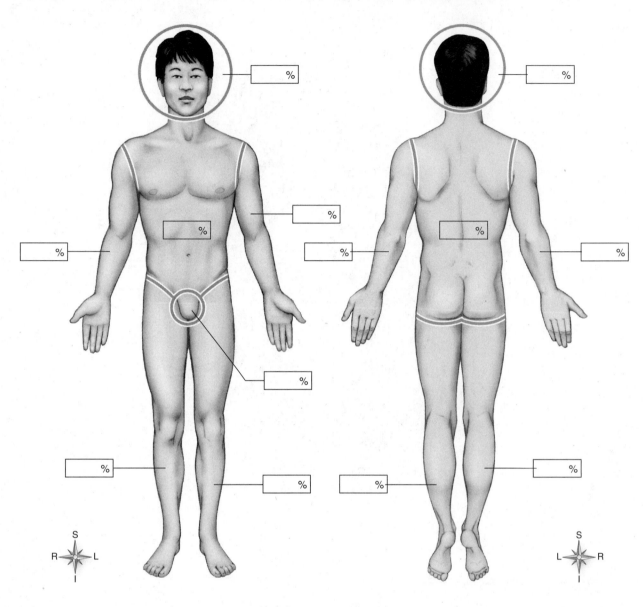

7
Skeletal System

How strange we would look without our skeleton! It is the skeleton that provides us with the rigid, supportive framework that gives shape to our bodies. But this is just the beginning, since it also protects the organs beneath it, maintains homeostasis of blood calcium, produces blood cells, and assists the muscular system in providing movement for us.

After reviewing the microscopic structure of bone and cartilage, you will understand how skeletal tissues are formed, their differences, and their importance in the human body. Your microscopic investigation will make the study of this system easier as you logically progress from this view to macroscopic bone formation and growth and visualize the structure of the long bones.

The skeleton is divided into two main divisions: the axial skeleton and the appendicular skeleton. All of the 206 bones of the human body may be classified into one of these two categories. And although we can divide the bones neatly by this system, we are still aware that subtle differences exist between men's and women's skeletons. These structural differences provide us with insight into the differences in function between men and women.

Finally, three types of joints exist in the body: synarthroses, amphiarthroses, and diarthroses. It is important to have knowledge of these joints and to understand how movement is facilitated by these various articulations.

TOPICS FOR REVIEW

Before progressing to Chapter 8, you should familiarize yourself with the functions of the skeletal system, the structure and function of bone and cartilage, bone formation and growth, and the types of joints found in the body. Additionally, your understanding of the skeletal system should enable you to identify the two major subdivisions of the skeleton, the bones found in each area, and any differences that exist between men's and women's skeletons.

FUNCTIONS OF THE SKELETAL SYSTEM—TYPES OF BONES

Fill in the blanks.

1. There are _____ types of bones.

2. The _____ _____ is the hollow area inside the diaphysis of a bone.

3. A thin layer of cartilage covering each epiphysis is the _____ _____.

4. The _____ lines the medullary cavity of long bones.

5. _____ is used to describe the process of blood cell formation.

6. Blood cell formation is a vital process carried on in _____ _____ _____.

7. The _____ is a strong fibrous membrane covering a long bone except at joint surfaces.

8. Osteoporosis occurs most frequently in _____ _____ _____.

9. Bones serve as a safety-deposit box for _____, a vital substance required for normal nerve and muscle function.

10. As muscles contract and shorten, they pull on bones and thereby _____ them.

➔ *If you had difficulty with this section, review pages 122-125 and 129.*

MICROSCOPIC STRUCTURE OF BONE AND CARTILAGE

Match the term on the left with the proper selection on the right.

Group A

11. _____ Trabeculae
12. _____ Compact
13. _____ Spongy
14. _____ Periosteum
15. _____ Cartilage

a. Outer covering of bone
b. Dense bone tissue
c. Fibers embedded in a firm gel
d. Needlelike threads of spongy bone
e. Porous bone

Group B

16. _____ Osteocytes
17. _____ Canaliculi
18. _____ Lamellae
19. _____ Chondrocytes
20. _____ Haversian system

a. Connect lacunae
b. Cartilage cells
c. Structural unit of compact bone
d. Bone cells
e. Ring of bone

➜ *If you had difficulty with this section, review page 125.*

BONE DEVELOPMENT

True or False

If the statement is true, write "T" in the answer blank. If the statement is false, correct the statement by circling the incorrect term and inserting the correct term in the answer blank.

21. _____ When the skeleton forms in a baby before birth, it consists of cartilage and fibrous structures.

22. _____ The diaphyses are the ends of the bone.

23. _____ Bone-forming cells are known as osteoclasts.

24. _____ It is the combined action of osteoblasts and osteoclasts that sculpts bones into their adult shapes.

25. _____ The stresses placed on certain bones during exercise decrease the rate of bone deposition.

26. _____ The epiphyseal plate can be seen in both external and cutaway views of an adult long bone.

27. _____ The shaft of a long bone is known as the articulation.

28. _____ Cartilage in the newborn becomes bone when it is replaced with calcified bone matrix deposited by osteoblasts.

29. _____ When epiphyseal cartilage becomes bone, growth begins.

30. _____ The epiphyseal cartilage is visible, if present, on x-ray films.

➜ *If you had difficulty with this section, review pages 127-128.*

AXIAL SKELETON AND APPENDICULAR SKELETON
Multiple Choice
Select the best answer.

31. Which one of the following is *not* a part of the axial skeleton?
   a. Scapula
   b. Cranial bones
   c. Vertebra
   d. Ribs
   e. Sternum

32. Which one of the following is *not* a cranial bone?
   a. Frontal
   b. Parietal
   c. Occipital
   d. Lacrimal
   e. Sphenoid

33. Which of the following statements is *not* true?
   a. A baby is born with a straight spine.
   b. In the adult, the sacral and thoracic curves are convex.
   c. The normal curves of the adult spine provide greater strength than a straight spine.
   d. A curved structure has more strength than a straight one of the same size and materials.

34. True ribs:
   a. Attach to the cartilage of other ribs
   b. Do not attach to the sternum
   c. Attach directly to the sternum without cartilage
   d. Attach directly to the sternum by means of cartilage

35. The bone that runs along the lateral side of your forearm is the:
   a. Humerus
   b. Ulna
   c. Radius
   d. Tibia

36. The shin bone is also known as the:
   a. Fibula
   b. Femur
   c. Tibia
   d. Ulna

37. The bones in the palm of the hand are called:
   a. Metatarsals
   b. Tarsals
   c. Carpals
   d. Metacarpals

38. Which one of the following is *not* a bone of the upper extremity?
   a. Radius
   b. Clavicle
   c. Humerus
   d. Ilium

39. The heel bone is known as the:
   a. Calcaneus
   b. Talus
   c. Metatarsal
   d. Phalanges

40. The mastoid process is part of the _____ bone.
    a. Parietal
    b. Temporal
    c. Occipital
    d. Frontal

41. When a baby learns to stand, the _____ area of the spine becomes concave.
    a. Lumbar
    b. Thoracic
    c. Cervical
    d. Coccyx

42. Which bone is the "funny" bone?
    a. Radius
    b. Ulna
    c. Humerus
    d. Carpal

43. There are _____ pairs of true ribs.
    a. 14
    b. 7
    c. 5
    d. 3

44. The 27 bones in the wrist and the hand allow for more:
    a. Strength
    b. Dexterity
    c. Protection
    d. Red blood cell production

45. The longest bone in the body is the:
    a. Tibia
    b. Fibula
    c. Femur
    d. Humerus

46. Distally, the _____ articulates with the patella.
    a. Femur
    b. Fibula
    c. Tibia
    d. Humerus

47. The _____ bones form the cheekbones.
    a. Mandible
    b. Palatine
    c. Maxillary
    d. Zygomatic

48. In a child, there are five of these bones. In an adult, they are fused into one.
    a. Pelvic
    b. Lumbar vertebrae
    c. Sacrum
    d. Carpals

49. The spinal cord enters the cranium through a large hole (foramen magnum) in the _____ bone.
    a. Temporal
    b. Parietal
    c. Occipital
    d. Sphenoid

Circle the one that does **not** *belong.*

50. Cervical   Thoracic   Coxal   Coccyx

51. Pelvic girdle   Ankle   Wrist   Axial

52. Frontal   Occipital   Maxilla   Sphenoid

53. Scapula   Pectoral girdle Ribs   Clavicle

54. Malleus   Vomer   Incus   Stapes

55. Ulna   Ilium   Ischium   Pubis

56. Carpal   Phalanges   Metacarpal   Ethmoid

57. Ethmoid   Parietal   Occipital   Nasal

58. Anvil   Atlas   Axis   Cervical

➔ *If you had difficulty with this section, review pages 128-141.*

SKELETAL VARIATIONS

Choose the correct answer.

a. Male
b. Female

59. _____ Funnel-shaped pelvis

60. _____ Broader-shaped pelvis

61. _____ Osteoporosis occurs more frequently

62. _____ Larger overall bone structure

63. _____ Wider pelvic inlet

➔ *If you had difficulty with this section, review pages 129 and 141.*

BONE MARKINGS

From the choices given, match the bone with the identifying marking. There may be more than one marking for some of the bones.

64. _____ Occipital

65. _____ Sternum

66. _____ Coxal

67. _____ Femur

68. _____ Ulna

69. _____ Temporal

70. _____ Tarsals

71. _____ Sphenoid

72. _____ Ethmoid

73. _____ Scapula

74. _____ Tibia

75. _____ Frontal

76. _____ Mandible

a. Mastoid
b. Pterygoid process
c. Foramen magnum
d. Sella turcica
e. Mental foramen
f. Conchae
g. Xiphoid process
h. Glenoid cavity
i. Olecranon process
j. Ischium
k. Acetabulum
l. Symphysis pubis
m. Ilium
n. Greater trochanter
o. Medial malleolus
p. Calcaneus
q. Acromion process
r. Frontal sinuses
s. Condyloid process
t. Tibial tuberosity

➔ *If you had difficulty with this section, review pages 131-140.*

JOINTS (ARTICULATIONS)

Circle the correct answer.

77. Freely movable joints are (*amphiarthroses* or *diarthroses*).

78. The sutures in the skull are (*synarthrotic* or *amphiarthrotic*) joints.

79. All (*diarthrotic* or *amphiarthrotic*) joints have a joint capsule, a joint cavity, and a layer of cartilage over the ends of the two joining bones.

80. (*Ligaments* or *tendons*) grow out of periosteum and attach two bones together.

81. The (*articular cartilage* or *epiphyseal cartilage*) absorbs jolts.

82. Gliding joints are the (*least* or *most*) movable of the diarthrotic joints.

83. The knee is the (*largest* or *smallest*) joint.

84. Hinge joints allow motion in (*2* or *4*) directions.

85. The saddle joint at the base of each of our thumbs allows for greater (*strength* or *mobility*).

86. When you rotate your head, you are using a (*gliding* or *pivot*) joint.

➡ *If you had difficulty with this section, review pages 143-147.*

UNSCRAMBLE THE BONES

Unscramble the circled letters and fill in the statement.

87. **E T V E R R B A E**

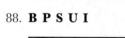

88. **B P S U I**

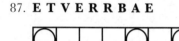

89. **S C A L U P A**

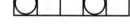

90. **I M D B A L N E**

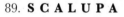

91. **A P N H G A E L S**

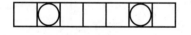

What the fat lady wore to the ball.

92.

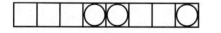

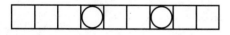

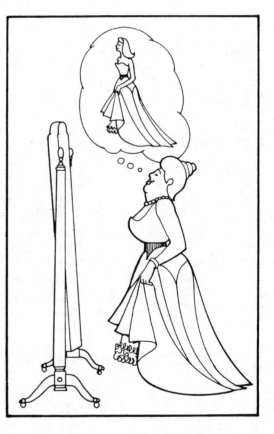

APPLYING WHAT YOU KNOW

93. Mrs. Perine had advanced cancer of the bone. As the disease progressed, Mrs. Perine required several blood transfusions throughout her therapy. One day she asked the doctor to explain the reason for the transfusions. What explanation might the doctor give to Mrs. Perine?

94. Dr. Kennedy, an orthopedic surgeon, called the admissions office of the hospital to advise that within the next hour he would be admitting a patient with an epiphyseal fracture. Without any other information, the patient is assigned to the pediatric ward. What prompted this assignment?

95. Mrs. Van Skiver, age 70, noticed when she went in for her physical examination that she was a half-inch shorter than she had been on her last visit. Dr. Veazey suggested she begin a regimen of calcium and vitamin D dietary supplements. Which bone disease did Dr. Veazey suspect?

96. While excavating a large section of land, workers found some bones that appeared to be the leg of a human. The coroner came back with a report stating that the bones were part of an adult male skeleton. How was he able to determine this information from a leg?

97. WORD FIND

Can you find 14 terms from this chapter in the box of letters? Words may be spelled top to bottom, bottom to top, right to left, left to right, or diagonally.

```
A  R  T  I  C  U  L  A  T  I  O  N  N  U  T
M  M  L  T  N  I  N  G  U  I  H  J  N  C  G
P  R  P  E  R  I  O  S  T  E  U  M  A  N  B
H  V  P  G  U  A  T  B  M  E  O  P  R  F  G
I  N  V  R  N  O  B  O  F  S  M  H  X  E  R
A  G  J  O  A  J  P  E  T  O  E  O  H  T  Q
R  U  R  B  X  O  E  E  C  A  S  G  I  S  B
T  S  S  Y  I  M  O  Q  N  U  O  O  L  X  Q
H  J  I  E  A  B  P  U  N  Q  L  E  Q  K  S
R  I  S  I  L  U  C  I  L  A  N  A  C  X  R
O  I  N  A  M  A  S  Q  M  A  Q  K  E  C  T
S  T  S  A  L  C  O  E  T  S  O  U  I  D  G
E  T  S  Y  F  W  L  N  M  P  U  F  N  U  F
S  B  H  Q  H  L  O  U  S  A  R  X  I  T  V
R  P  M  P  A  F  M  G  X  K  D  S  L  G  A
```

Amphiarthroses	Fontanels	Osteoclasts
Articulation	Hemopoiesis	Periosteum
Axial	Lacunae	Sinus
Canaliculi	Lamella	Trabeculae
Compact	Osteoblasts	

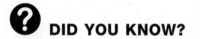

DID YOU KNOW?

- The bones of the hands and feet make up more than half of the total 206 bones of the body.
- The size of your foot is approximately the size of your forearm.
- The average person flexes his or her finger joints 25 million times during a lifetime.
- Babies are born with 300 bones, but by adulthood we have only 206 in our bodies.
- The bones of the middle ear are mature at birth.

SKELETAL SYSTEM

Fill in the crossword puzzle.

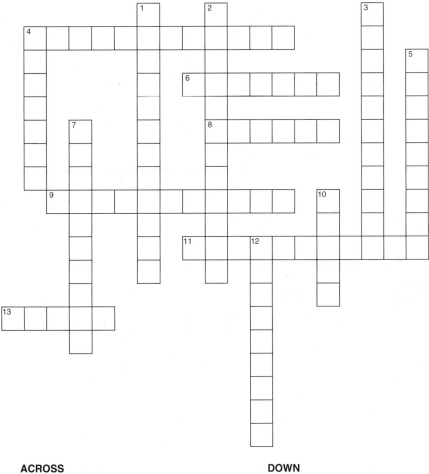

ACROSS
4. Cartilage cells
6. Spaces in bones where osteocytes are found
8. Chest
9. Freely movable joints
11. Process of blood cell formation
13. Space inside cranial bone

DOWN
1. Joint
2. Suture joints
3. Bone absorbing cells
4. Type of bone
5. Ends of long bones
7. Covers long bone except at its joint surfaces
10. Division of skeleton
12. Bone cell

CHECK YOUR KNOWLEDGE

Multiple Choice

Select the best answer.

1. Which of the following is *not* a function of bones?
   a. Communication
   b. Storage
   c. Hematopoiesis
   d. Protection

2. The four types of bones are:
   a. Flat, irregular, short, and square
   b. Flat, cartilage, short, and long
   c. Flat, irregular, short, and long
   d. Small, long, flat, and heavy

3. Which of the following is *not* a main part of a long bone?
   a. Malleus
   b. Epiphyses
   c. Periosteum
   d. Diaphysis

4. All of the following bones are part of the appendicular skeleton *except:*
   a. Shoulder
   b. Hip
   c. Chest
   d. Feet

5. There are a total of _____ phalanges in the skeletal system.
   a. 28
   b. 60
   c. 56
   d. 72

6. Cartilage differs from bone because it:
   a. Is embedded in a firm gel rather than in a calcified cement substance
   b. Has the flexibility of a firm plastic rather than being rigid
   c. Rebuilds itself very slowly after injury
   d. All of the above

7. Which of the following is *not* a paranasal sinus?
   a. Frontal
   b. Ethmoid
   c. Lambdoidal
   d. Sphenoid

8. The last two ribs:
   a. Attach directly to the sternum
   b. Are attached to costal cartilage
   c. Are referred to as "floating ribs"
   d. None of the above

9. In an infant, each coxal bone consists of three separate bones. These bones are the:
   a. Ilium, ischium, and coccyx
   b. Ischium, pubis, and tuberosity
   c. Pubis, tuberosity, and coccyx
   d. Ilium, ischium, and pubis

10. An example of a synarthrotic joint is:
    a. A cranial suture
    b. The hip joint
    c. The shoulder joint
    d. The spine

Matching

Select the most correct answer from column B for each statement in column A. (Only one answer is correct.)

Column A

11. _____ Articulation

12. _____ Medullary cavity

13. _____ Osteons

14. _____ Incus

15. _____ Sternum

16. _____ Zygomatic

17. _____ Olecranon process

18. _____ Synarthroses

19. _____ Hinge joint

20. _____ Thumb joint

Column B

a. "Funny bone"
b. Yellow bone marrow
c. Immovable
d. Circumduct
e. Manubrium
f. Flexion
g. Joint
h. Cheekbone
i. Haversian system
j. Middle ear

LONGITUDINAL SECTION OF LONG BONE

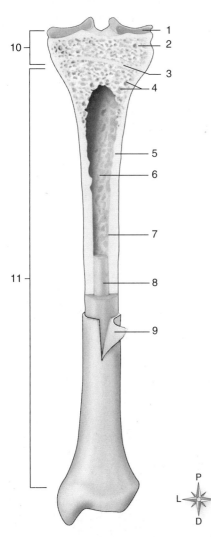

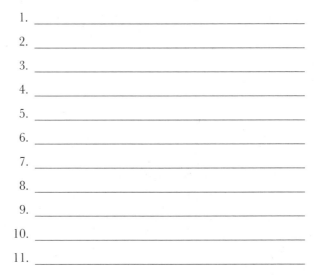

1. _____

2. _____

3. _____

4. _____

5. _____

6. _____

7. _____

8. _____

9. _____

10. _____

11. _____

ANTERIOR VIEW OF SKELETON

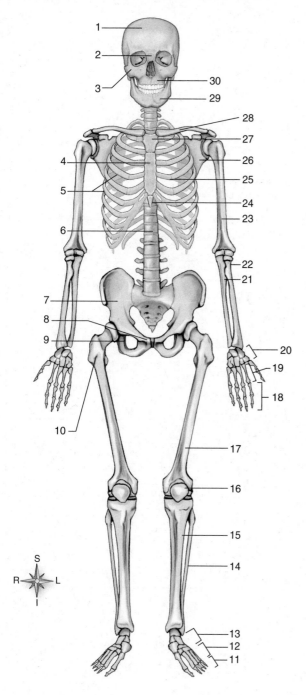

1. _____

2. _____

3. _____

4. _____

5. _____

6. _____

7. _____

8. _____

9. _____

10. _____

11. _____

12. _____

13. _____

14. _____

15. _____

16. _____

17. _____

18. _____

19. _____

20. _____

21. _____

22. _____

23. _____

24. _____

25. _____

26. _____

27. _____

28. _____

29. _____

30. _____

POSTERIOR VIEW OF SKELETON

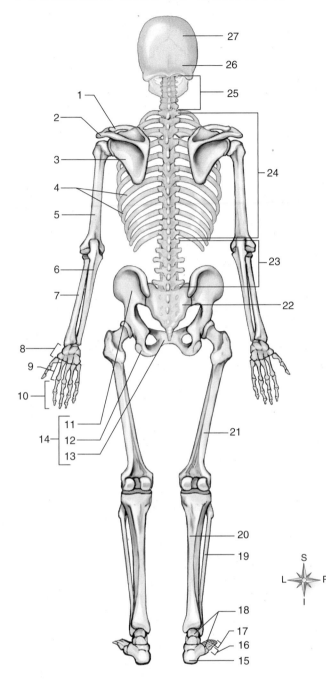

1. _____
2. _____
3. _____
4. _____
5. _____
6. _____
7. _____
8. _____
9. _____
10. _____
11. _____
12. _____
13. _____
14. _____
15. _____
16. _____
17. _____
18. _____
19. _____
20. _____
21. _____
22. _____
23. _____
24. _____
25. _____
26. _____
27. _____

SKULL VIEWED FROM THE RIGHT SIDE

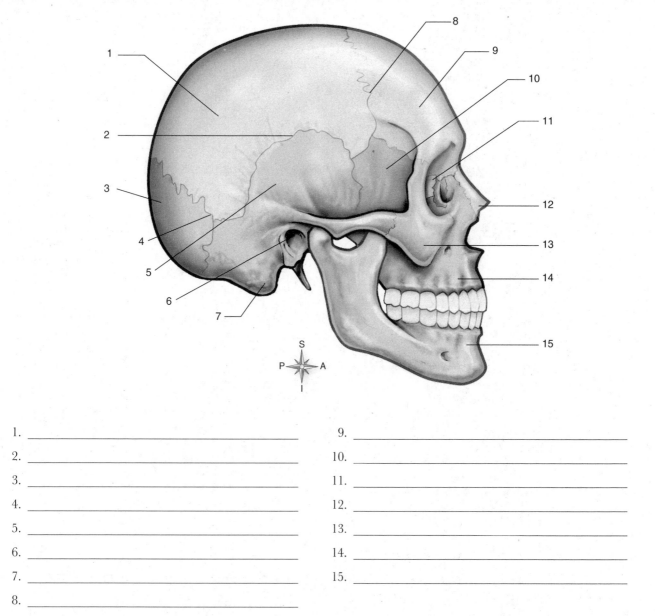

1. _____

2. _____

3. _____

4. _____

5. _____

6. _____

7. _____

8. _____

9. _____

10. _____

11. _____

12. _____

13. _____

14. _____

15. _____

SKULL VIEWED FROM THE FRONT

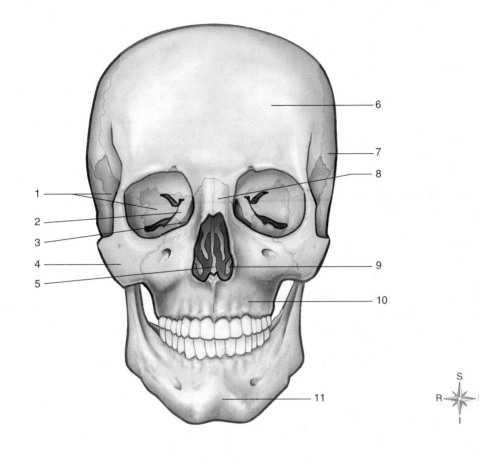

1. _____

2. _____

3. _____

4. _____

5. _____

6. _____

7. _____

8. _____

9. _____

10. _____

11. _____

STRUCTURE OF A DIARTHROTIC JOINT

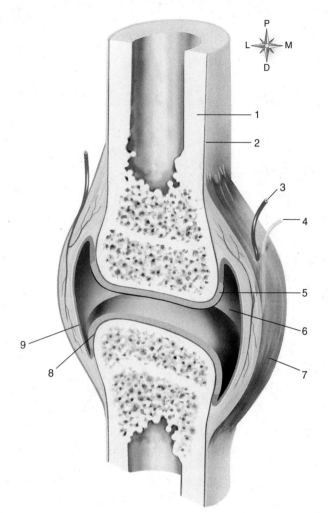

1. _____
2. _____
3. _____
4. _____
5. _____
6. _____
7. _____
8. _____
9. _____

CHAPTER 8

Muscular System

The muscular system is often referred to as the *power system*, and rightfully so, because it is this system that provides the force necessary to move the body and perform organic functions. Just as an automobile relies on the engine to provide motion, the body depends on the muscular system to perform both voluntary and involuntary types of movements. Walking, breathing, and the digestion of food are but a few examples of body functions that require the healthy performance of the muscular system.

Although this system has several functions, the primary purpose is to provide movement or power. Muscles produce power by contracting. The ability of a large muscle or muscle group to contract depends on the ability of microscopic muscle fibers that contract within the larger muscle. An understanding of these microscopic muscle fibers will assist you as your study progresses to the larger muscles and muscle groups.

Muscle contractions may be one of several types: isotonic, isometric, twitch, or tetanic. When skeletal or voluntary muscles contract, they provide us with a variety of motions. Flexion, extension, abduction, adduction, and rotation are examples of these movements that provide us with both strength and agility.

Muscles must be used to keep the body healthy and in good condition. Scientific evidence keeps pointing to the fact that the proper use and exercise of muscles may extend longevity. An understanding of the structure and function of the muscular system may, therefore, add quality and quantity to our lives.

TOPICS FOR REVIEW

Before progressing to Chapter 9, you should familiarize yourself with the structure and function of the three major types of muscle tissues. Your review should include the microscopic structure of skeletal muscle tissue, the mechanism by which a muscle is stimulated, the major types of skeletal muscle contractions, and the skeletal muscle groups. Your study should conclude with an understanding of the types of movements produced by skeletal muscle contractions.

MUSCLE TISSUE

Select the correct term(s) from the choices given and write the letter in the answer blank.

a. Skeletal muscle
b. Cardiac muscle
c. Smooth muscle

1. _____ Striated
2. _____ Cells branch frequently
3. _____ Moves food into stomach
4. _____ Nonstriated
5. _____ Voluntary
6. _____ Increases efficiency of heart muscle in pumping blood
7. _____ Involuntary
8. _____ Attaches to bone
9. _____ Found in hollow internal organs
10. _____ Also called *visceral muscle*

➡ *If you had difficulty with this section, review pages 154-156.*

STRUCTURE OF SKELETAL MUSCLE

Match the term on the left with the proper selection on the right.

Group A

11. _____ Origin

12. _____ Insertion

13. _____ Body

14. _____ Tendons

15. _____ Bursae

a. The muscle unit, excluding the ends
b. Attachment to the more movable bone
c. Fluid-filled sacs
d. Attachment to more stationary bone
e. Attach muscle to bones

Group B

16. _____ Muscle fibers

17. _____ Actin

18. _____ Sarcomere

19. _____ Myosin

20. _____ Myofilament

a. Protein that forms thick myofilaments
b. Basic functional unit of skeletal muscle
c. Protein that forms thin myofilaments
d. Microscopic threadlike structures found in skeletal muscle fibers
e. Elongated contractile cells of muscle tissue

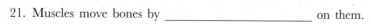 *If you had difficulty with this section, review pages 156-159.*

FUNCTIONS OF SKELETAL MUSCLE

Fill in the blanks.

21. Muscles move bones by _____ on them.

22. As a rule, only the _____ bone moves.

23. The _____ bone moves toward the _____ bone.

24. Of all the muscles contracting simultaneously, the one mainly responsible for producing a particular movement is called the _____ _____ for that movement.

25. As prime movers contract, muscles called _____ relax.

26. The biceps brachii is the prime mover during bending, and the brachialis is its helper or _____ muscle.

27. We are able to maintain our body position because of a specialized type of skeletal muscle contraction called _____ _____.

28. _____ _____ maintains body posture by counteracting the pull of gravity.

29. A decrease in temperature, a condition known as _____, will dramatically affect cellular activity and normal body function.

30. Energy required to produce a muscle contraction is obtained from _____.

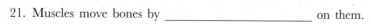 *If you had difficulty with this section, review pages 159-160.*

MUSCLE FATIGUE—ROLE OF BODY SYSTEMS IN MOVEMENT—MOTOR UNIT—MUSCLE STIMULUS

True or False

If the statement is true, write "T" in the answer blank. If the statement is false, correct the statement by circling the incorrect term and writing the correct term in the answer blank.

31. _____ The point of contact between the nerve ending and the muscle fiber is called a motor neuron.

32. _____ A motor neuron together with the cells it innervates is called a motor unit.

33. _____ If muscle cells are stimulated repeatedly without adequate periods of rest, the strength of the muscle contraction will decrease, resulting in fatigue.

34. _____ The depletion of oxygen in muscle cells during vigorous and prolonged exercise is known as fatigue.

35. _____ An adequate stimulus will contract a muscle cell completely because of the "must" theory.

36. _____ When oxygen supplies run low, muscle cells produce ATP and other waste products during contraction.

37. _____ In a laboratory setting, a single muscle fiber can be isolated and subjected to stimuli of varying intensities so that it can be studied.

38. _____ The minimal level of stimulation required to cause a fiber to contract is called the threshold stimulus.

39. _____ Smooth muscles bring about movements by pulling on bones across movable joints.

40. _____ A nervous system disorder that shuts off impulses to certain skeletal muscles may result in paralysis.

TYPES OF SKELETAL MUSCLE CONTRACTIONS

Select the best answer.

41. When a muscle does not shorten and no movement results, the contraction is:
    a. Isometric
    b. Isotonic
    c. Twitch
    d. Tetanic

42. Walking is an example of which type of contraction?
    a. Isometric
    b. Isotonic
    c. Twitch
    d. Tetanic

43. Pushing against a wall is an example of which type of contraction?
    a. Isotonic
    b. Isometric
    c. Twitch
    d. Tetanic

44. Endurance training is also known as:
    a. Isometrics
    b. Hypertrophy
    c. Aerobic training
    d. Strength training

45. Benefits of regular exercise include all of the following *except:*
    a. Improved lung function
    b. More efficient heart
    c. Less fatigue
    d. Atrophy

46. Twitch contractions can be easily seen in:
    a. Isolated muscles prepared for research
    b. A great deal of normal muscle activity
    c. During resting periods
    d. None of the above

47. Contractions that "melt" together to produce a sustained contraction are called:
    a. Twitch
    b. Tetanus
    c. Isotonic response
    d. Isometric response

48. In most cases, isotonic contraction of muscle produces movement at a(n):
    a. Insertion
    b. Origin
    c. Joint
    d. Bursa

49. Prolonged inactivity causes muscles to shrink in mass, producing a condition called:
    a. Hypertrophy
    b. Disuse atrophy
    c. Paralysis
    d. Muscle fatigue

50. Muscle hypertrophy can be best enhanced by a program of:
    a. Isotonic exercise
    b. Better posture
    c. High-protein diet
    d. Strength training

➙ *If you had difficulty with this section, review pages 160-164.*

MOVEMENTS PRODUCED BY SKELETAL MUSCLE CONTRACTIONS

Select the best answer.

51. A movement that makes the angle between two bones smaller is:
    a. Flexion
    b. Extension
    c. Abduction
    d. Adduction

52. Moving a part toward the midline is:
    a. Flexion
    b. Extension
    c. Abduction
    d. Adduction

53. Moving a part away from the midline is:
    a. Flexion
    b. Extension
    c. Abduction
    d. Adduction

54. When you move your head from side to side as in shaking your head "no," you are _____ a muscle group.
    a. Rotating
    b. Pronating
    c. Supinating
    d. Abducting

55. _____ occurs when you turn the palm of your hand from an anterior to posterior position.
    a. Dorsiflexion
    b. Plantar flexion
    c. Supination
    d. Pronation

56. *Dorsiflexion* refers to:
    a. Hand movements
    b. Eye movements
    c. Foot movements
    d. Head movements

➡ *If you had difficulty with this section, review pages 164-167.*

SKELETAL MUSCLE GROUPS

Choose the proper function or functions for the muscles listed below and write the appropriate letter or letters in the answer blank.

a. Flexor
b. Extensor
c. Abductor
d. Adductor
e. Rotator
f. Dorsiflexor or plantar flexor

57. _____ Deltoid

58. _____ Tibialis anterior

59. _____ Gastrocnemius

60. _____ Biceps brachii

61. _____ Gluteus medius

62. _____ Soleus

63. _____ Iliopsoas

64. _____ Pectoralis major

65. _____ Gluteus maximus

66. _____ Triceps brachii

67. _____ Sternocleidomastoid

68. _____ Trapezius

69. _____ Gracilis

➡ *If you had difficulty with this section, review pages 167-172.*

UNSCRAMBLE THE WORD

Unscramble the circled letters and fill in the statement.

70. **N F O X L I E**

☐ ☐ ☐ Ⓞ ☐ ☐ ☐

71. **T N I C A**

☐ Ⓞ ☐ Ⓞ ☐

72. **V R S N E I O E**

☐ ☐ ☐ Ⓞ ☐ ☐ Ⓞ

73. **I O R N I G**

Ⓞ ☐ ☐ Ⓞ ☐ ☐

74. **S E A R R E C M O**

☐ ☐ ☐ ☐ ☐ Ⓞ ☐ Ⓞ

What Kevin requested for his IOU.

75.

☐ ☐ ☐ ☐ ☐ ☐ ☐ ☐ ☐

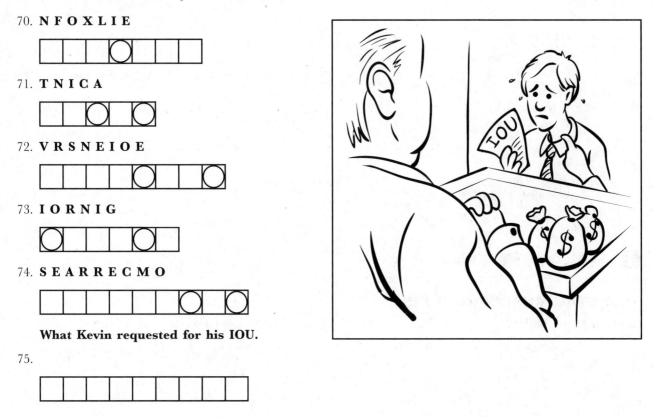

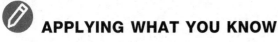

APPLYING WHAT YOU KNOW

76. Casey noticed pain whenever she reached for anything in her cupboards. Her doctor told her that the small fluid-filled sacs in her shoulder were inflamed. What condition did Casey have?

77. Ed spends hours typing on his computer. Lately, he has been experiencing weakness, pain, and tingling in the palm and radial aspect of his hand. What condition may he be experiencing? Which anatomical structures are most likely involved with this condition? What options for treatment are available?

78. Chris was playing football and pulled a band of fibrous connective tissue that attached a muscle to a bone. What is the common term for this tissue?

79. WORD FIND

Can you find the 25 muscle terms in the box of letters? Words may be spelled top to bottom, bottom to top, right to left, left to right, or diagonally.

```
G A S T R O C N E M I U S D U
M S G I O N O I S N E T X E U
U R N N T O M S R B S F D T T
S U I S C I B O N T P N E A R
C B R E U X V T O O E C L I A
L Q T R D E C O D A C M T R P
E T S T B L M N N V I E O T E
X F M I A F Y I E Y B N I S Z
S I A O V I E C T L S S D I I
S Y H N S S R O T A T O R G U
U A M G A R H P A I D J N R S
E H A T R O P H Y L N J T E B
L N O H T D E U G I T A F N T
O R I G I N O S N V S B Z Y L
S B V T O J C T R I C E P S S
```

Abductor	Extension	Isometric	Striated
Atrophy	Fatigue	Isotonic	Synergist
Biceps	Flexion	Muscle	Tendon
Bursa	Gastrocnemius	Origin	Tenosynovitis
Deltoid	Hamstrings	Rotator	Trapezius
Diaphragm	Insertion	Soleus	Triceps
Dorsiflexion			

❓ DID YOU KNOW?

- If all of your muscles pulled in one direction, you would have the power to move 25 tons.
- The simple act of walking requires the use of 200 muscles in the human body.
- A cat has 32 muscles in each ear.

THE MUSCULAR SYSTEM

Fill in the crossword puzzle.

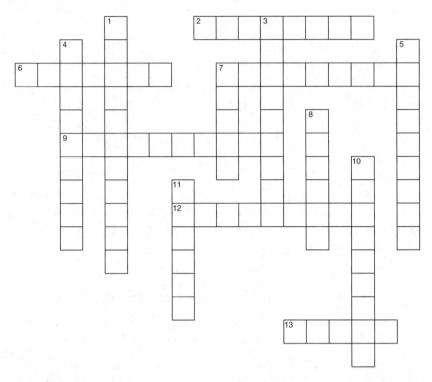

ACROSS

2. Shaking your head "no"
6. Muscle shrinkage
7. Toward the body's midline
9. Produces movement opposite to prime movers
12. Movement that makes joint angles larger
13. Small fluid-filled sac between tendons and bones

DOWN

1. Increase in size
3. Away from the body's midline
4. Turning your palm from an anterior to posterior position
5. Attachment to the more movable bone
7. Protein that composes myofilaments
8. Attachment to the more stationary bone
10. Assists prime movers with movement
11. Anchors muscles to bones

CHECK YOUR KNOWLEDGE

Multiple Choice

Select the best answer.

1. Endurance training is also called:
   a. Isometrics
   b. Hypertrophy
   c. Anaerobic training
   d. Aerobic training

2. Increase in muscle size is called:
   a. Hypertrophy
   b. Atrophy
   c. Hyperplasia
   d. Treppe

3. Which of the following statements concerning isometric contractions is true?
   a. Walking is an example of an isometric contraction.
   b. Muscle tension decreases.
   c. Muscle length remains constant.
   d. Movement of the muscle increases.

4. Muscle cells are stimulated by a nerve fiber called a:
   a. Sarcomere
   b. Motor neuron
   c. Myofilament
   d. Prime mover

5. Muscles that help other muscles produce movement are called:
   a. Synergists
   b. Prime movers
   c. Antagonists
   d. None of the above

6. The connecting bridges between myofilaments form properly only if _____ is present.
   a. Potassium
   b. Calcium
   c. Sodium
   d. Chloride

7. Physiological muscle fatigue is caused by:
   a. Oxygen debt
   b. Inadequate periods of rest for muscles
   c. Lactic acid buildup in the muscles
   d. All of the above

8. The muscle's attachment to the more stationary bone is called its:
   a. Origin
   b. Body
   c. Insertion
   d. None of the above

9. Skeletal muscle:
   a. Is voluntary
   b. Is smooth
   c. Is also known as *visceral muscle*
   d. All of the above

10. Which of the following is *not* a hamstring muscle?
    a. Semimembranosus
    b. Semitendinosus
    c. Rectus femoris
    d. Biceps femoris

True or False

If the statement is true, write "T" in the answer blank. If the statement is false, correct the statement by circling the incorrect term and writing the correct term in the answer blank.

11. _____ The "all or none" principle states that when a muscle fiber is subjected to a threshold stimulus, it contracts completely.

12. _____ Muscle tone maintains posture.

13. _____ Thick myofilaments are formed from a protein called *actin*.

14. _____ The triceps brachii is on the anterior surface of the upper arm.

15. _____ Tendons anchor muscles firmly to bones.

16. _____ Energy required to produce a muscle contraction is obtained from ATP.

17. _____ Rotation is movement around a longitudinal axis.

18. _____ Extension movements are the opposite of abduction.

19. _____ The gastrocnemius is responsible for plantar flexion of the foot and is sometimes referred to as the *toe dancer's muscle*.

20. _____ An explanation of how a skeletal muscle contracts is provided by the sliding filament model.

MUSCLES—ANTERIOR VIEW

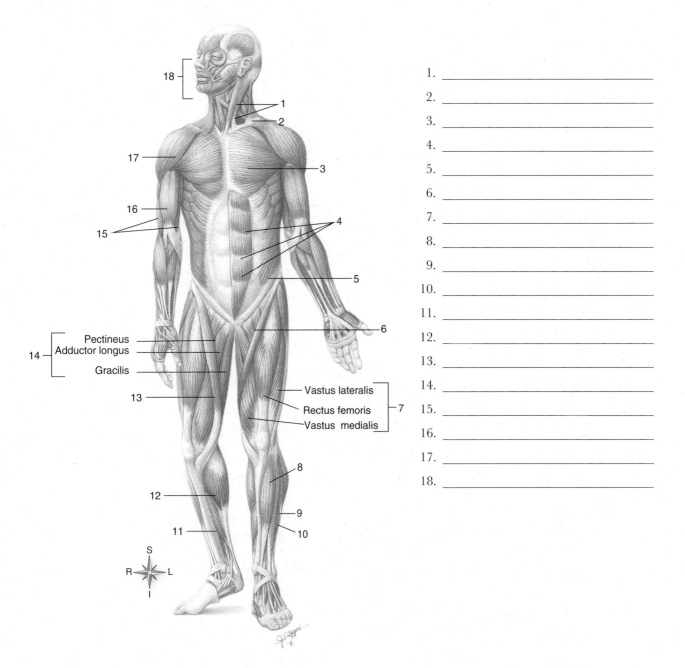

1. _____

2. _____

3. _____

4. _____

5. _____

6. _____

7. _____

8. _____

9. _____

10. _____

11. _____

12. _____

13. _____

14. _____

15. _____

16. _____

17. _____

18. _____

MUSCLES—POSTERIOR VIEW

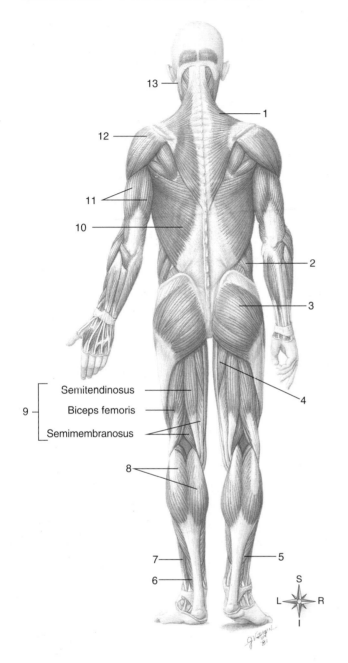

Semitendinosus

Biceps femoris

Semimembranosus

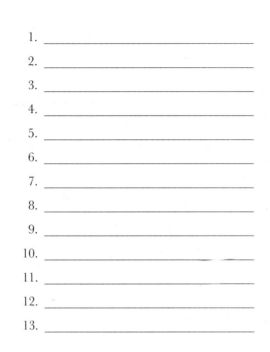

1. _____
2. _____
3. _____
4. _____
5. _____
6. _____
7. _____
8. _____
9. _____
10. _____
11. _____
12. _____
13. _____

Nervous System

The nervous system organizes and coordinates the millions of impulses received each day to make communication with and enjoyment of our environment possible. The functioning unit of the nervous system is the neuron. Three types of neurons—sensory neurons, motor neurons, and interneurons—exist and are classified according to the direction in which they transmit impulses. Nerve impulses travel over routes made up of neurons and provide the rapid communication necessary for maintaining life. The central nervous system is made up of the spinal cord and brain. The spinal cord provides access to and from the brain by means of ascending and descending tracts. In addition, the spinal cord functions as the primary reflex center of the body. The brain can be subdivided for easier learning into the brain stem, cerebellum, diencephalon, and cerebrum. These areas provide the extraordinary network necessary to receive, interpret, and respond to the simplest or most complex impulses.

The peripheral nervous system is the system of nerves connecting the brain and spinal cord to other parts of the body. These nerves, known as the *cranial* and *spinal nerves,* may be further divided into the autonomic (involuntary) nervous system and the somatic (voluntary) nervous system. Sensory nerves are also considered part of the peripheral nervous system. The sensory nerves form the link between receptors and the central nervous system (CNS). They carry nerve impulses from stimulated receptors to the CNS and are considered part of the peripheral nervous system.

While you concentrate on this chapter, your body is performing a multitude of functions. Fortunately for us, breathing, beating of the heart, digestion of food, and most of our other day-to-day processes do not require our supervision or thought. They function automatically, and the division of the nervous system that regulates these functions is known as the *autonomic nervous system.*

The autonomic nervous system may be further subdivided into two divisions called the *sympathetic system* and the *parasympathetic system.* The sympathetic system functions as an emergency system and prepares us for "fight or flight." The parasympathetic system dominates control of many visceral effectors under normal everyday conditions. Together, these two divisions regulate the body's automatic functions in an effort to assist with the maintenance of homeostasis. Your understanding of this chapter will alert you to the complexity and functions of the nervous system and the "automatic pilot" of your body—the autonomic system.

TOPICS FOR REVIEW

Before progressing to Chapter 10, you should review the organs and divisions of the nervous system, the structure and function of the major types of cells in this system, the structure and function of a reflex arc, and the transmission of nerve impulses. Your study should include the anatomy and physiology of the brain and spinal cord and the nerves that extend from these two areas.

Finally, an understanding of the autonomic nervous system and the specific functions of the subdivisions of this system are necessary to complete the review of this chapter.

ORGANIZATION OF THE NERVOUS SYSTEM—CELLS OF THE NERVOUS SYSTEM—NERVES AND TRACTS

Match the term on the left with the proper selection on the right.

Group A

1. _____ Sense organ
2. _____ Central nervous system
3. _____ Peripheral nervous system
4. _____ Autonomic nervous system

a. Subdivision of peripheral nervous system
b. Ear
c. Brain and spinal cord
d. Nerves that extend to the outlying parts of the body

Group B

5. _____ Dendrite

6. _____ Schwann cell

7. _____ Motor neuron

8. _____ Nodes of Ranvier

9. _____ Fascicles

10. _____ Epineurium

a. Gaps between adjacent Schwann cells
b. Branching projection of neuron
c. Also known as *efferent*
d. Forms myelin outside the central nervous system
e. Tough sheath that covers the whole nerve
f. Groups of wrapped axon

NEURONS/GLIA

Select the correct term from the choices given and write the letter in the answer blank.

a. Neurons
b. Neuroglia

11. _____ Axon

12. _____ Special type of supporting cells

13. _____ Astrocytes

14. _____ Sensory

15. _____ Conduct impulses

16. _____ Forms the myelin sheath around central nerve fibers

17. _____ Phagocytosis

18. _____ Efferent

19. _____ Multiple sclerosis

20. _____ Neurilemma

➔ *If you had difficulty with this section, review pages 179-182 and 184.*

NERVE SIGNALS—REFLEX ARCS

Fill in the blanks.

21. The simplest kind of reflex arc is a(n) _____ _____ _____.

22. Three-neuron arcs consist of all three kinds of neurons: _____, _____, and _____ _____.

23. Impulse conduction in a reflex arc normally starts in _____.

24. A(n) _____ is the place where impulses are transmitted from one neuron to another neuron.

25. A(n) _____ is the response to impulse conduction over reflex arcs.

26. Contraction of a muscle that causes it to pull away from an irritating stimulus is known as the _____ _____.

27. A(n) _____ is a group of nerve cell bodies located in the peripheral nervous system.

28. All _____ lie entirely within the gray matter of the central nervous system.

29. In a patellar reflex, the nerve impulses that reach the quadriceps muscle (the effector) result in the classic "_____ _____" response.

30. _____ _____ forms the H-shaped inner core of the spinal cord.

➔ *If you had difficulty with this section, review pages 182-184.*

NERVE IMPULSES—THE SYNAPSE

Circle the correct answer.

31. Nerve impulses (*do* or *do not*) continually race along every nerve cell's surface.

32. When a stimulus acts on a neuron, it (*increases* or *decreases*) the permeability of the stimulated point of its membrane to sodium ions.

33. An inward movement of positive ions leaves (*a lack* or *an excess*) of negative ions outside.

34. The plasma membrane of the (*presynaptic* or *postsynaptic*) neuron makes up a portion of the synapse.

35. A synaptic knob is a tiny bulge at the end of the (*presynaptic* or *postsynaptic*) neuron's axon.

36. Acetylcholine is an example of a (*neurotransmitter* or *protein molecule receptor*).

37. Neurotransmitters are chemicals that allow neurons to (*communicate* or *reproduce*) with one another.

38. Neurotransmitters are distributed (*randomly* or *specifically*) into groups of neurons.

39. Catecholamines may play a role in (*sleep* or *reproduction*).

40. Endorphins and enkephalins are neurotransmitters that inhibit conduction of (*fear* or *pain*) impulses.

➡ *If you had difficulty with this section, review pages 184-188.*

CENTRAL NERVOUS SYSTEM—BRAIN

Select the best answer.

41. Which one of the following is a part of the brainstem?
    a. Thalamus
    b. Cerebellum
    c. Cerebrum
    d. Hypothalamus
    e. Medulla

42. Which one of the following is *not* a function of the brainstem?
    a. Conduction of sensory impulses from the spinal cord to the higher centers of the brain
    b. Conduction of motor impulses from the cerebrum to the spinal cord
    c. Control of heartbeat, respiration, and blood vessel diameter
    d. Containment of centers for speech and memory

43. Which one of the following is *not* part of the diencephalon?
    a. Cerebrum
    b. Thalamus
    c. Hypothalamus
    d. All of the above are correct

44. ADH is produced by the:
    a. Pituitary gland
    b. Medulla
    c. Mammillary bodies
    d. Third ventricle
    e. Hypothalamus

45. Which one of the following is *not* true about the hypothalamus?
    a. It helps control the rate of heartbeat.
    b. It helps control the constriction and dilation of blood vessels.
    c. It helps control the contraction of the stomach and intestines.
    d. It produces releasing hormones that control the release of certain anterior pituitary hormones.
    e. All of the above are true.

46. Which one of the following parts of the brain helps in the association of sensations with emotions and also aids in the arousal or alerting mechanism?
    a. Pons
    b. Hypothalamus
    c. Cerebellum
    d. Thalamus
    e. None of the above

47. Which of the following is *not* true of the cerebrum?
    a. Its lobes correspond to the bones that lie over them.
    b. Its grooves are called *gyri.*
    c. Most of its gray matter lies on the surface of the cerebrum.
    d. Its outer region is called the *cerebral cortex.*
    e. Its two hemispheres are connected by a structure called the *corpus callosum.*

48. Which one of the following is *not* a function of the cerebrum?
    a. Willed movement
    b. Consciousness
    c. Memory
    d. Conscious awareness of sensations
    e. All of the above are functions of the cerebrum

49. The area of the cerebrum responsible for the perception of sound lies in the _____ lobe.
    a. Frontal
    b. Temporal
    c. Occipital
    d. Parietal

50. Visual perception is located in the _____ lobe.
    a. Frontal
    b. Temporal
    c. Parietal
    d. Occipital
    e. None of the above

51. Which one of the following is *not* a function of the cerebellum?
    a. Maintains equilibrium
    b. Helps with production of smooth, coordinated movements
    c. Helps maintain normal posture
    d. Associates sensations with emotions

52. Within the interior of the cerebrum are a few islands of gray matter known as:
    a. Fissures
    b. Basal ganglia
    c. Gyri
    d. Myelin

53. A cerebrovascular accident is commonly referred to as:
    a. A stroke
    b. Parkinson's disease
    c. A tumor
    d. Multiple sclerosis

54. Parkinson's disease is a disease of the:
    a. Myelin
    b. Axons
    c. Neuroglia
    d. Cerebral basal nuclei

55. The largest section of the brain is the:
    a. Cerebellum
    b. Pons
    c. Cerebrum
    d. Midbrain

➡ *If you had difficulty with this section, review pages 188-192.*

SPINAL CORD

True or False

If the statement is true, write "T" in the answer blank. If the statement is false, correct the statement by circling the incorrect term and writing the correct term in the answer blank.

56. _____ The spinal cord is approximately 24-25 inches long.

57. _____ The spinal cord ends at the bottom of the sacrum.

58. _____ The extension of the meninges beyond the cord is convenient for performing CAT scans without danger of injuring the spinal cord.

59. _____ Bundles of myelinated nerve fibers (dendrites) make up the white outer columns of the spinal cord.

60. _____ Ascending tracts conduct impulses up the cord to the brain, and descending tracts conduct impulses down the cord from the brain.

61. _____ Tracts are functional organizations in that all the axons that compose a tract serve several functions.

62. _____ A loss of sensation caused by a spinal cord injury is called paralysis.

➡ *If you had difficulty with this section, review pages 193-194 and 197.*

COVERINGS AND FLUID SPACES OF THE BRAIN AND SPINAL CORD

Circle the one that does not belong.

63. Meninges	Pia mater	Ventricles	Dura mater
64. Arachnoid	Middle layer	CSF	Cobweb-like
65. CSF	Ventricles	Subarachnoid space	Pia mater
66. Tough	Outer layer	Dura mater	Choroid plexus
67. Brain tumor	Subarachnoid space	CSF	Fourth lumbar vertebra

➡ *If you had difficulty with this section, review pages 194-197.*

PERIPHERAL NERVOUS SYSTEM—CRANIAL NERVES

68. *Fill in the missing areas on the chart below.*

Nerve		Conduct Impulses	Function
I		From nose to brain	Sense of smell
II	Optic	From eye to brain	
III	Oculomotor		Eye movements
IV		From brain to external eye muscles	Eye movements
V	Trigeminal	From skin and mucous membrane of head and from teeth to brain, also from brain to chewing muscles	
VI	Abducens		Eye movements
VII	Facial	From taste buds of tongue to brain, from brain to face muscles	
VIII		From ear to brain	Hearing, sense of balance
IX	Glossopharyngeal		Sensations of throat, taste, swallowing movements, secretion of saliva
X		From throat, larynx, and organs in thoracic and abdominal cavities to brain; also from brain to muscles of throat and to organs in thoracic and abdominal cavities	Sensations of throat, larynx, and of thoracic and abdominal organs; swallowing; voice production; slowing of heartbeat;acceleration of peristalsis (gut movements)
XI	Accessory	From brain to certain shoulder and neck muscles	
XII		From brain to muscles of tongue	Tongue movements

➔ *If you had difficulty with this section, review page 197 and Table 9-2.*

PERIPHERAL NERVOUS SYSTEM—CRANIAL NERVES—SPINAL NERVES

Select the correct term from the choices given and write its letter in the answer blank.

a. Cranial nerves
b. Spinal nerves

69. _____ 12 pairs

70. _____ Dermatome

71. _____ Vagus

72. _____ Shingles

73. _____ 31 pairs

74. _____ Optic

75. _____ C1

76. _____ Plexus

➡️ *If you had difficulty with this section, review pages 197-199 and 203.*

AUTONOMIC NERVOUS SYSTEM

Match the term on the left with the proper selection on the right.

77. _____ Autonomic nervous system

78. _____ Autonomic neurons

79. _____ Preganglionic neurons

80. _____ Visceral effectors

81. _____ Sympathetic system

82. _____ Somatic nervous system

a. Division of ANS
b. Tissues to which autonomic neurons conduct impulses
c. Voluntary actions
d. Regulates body's involuntary functions
e. Motor neurons that make up the ANS
f. Conduct impulses between the spinal cord and a ganglion

FUNCTIONAL ANATOMY—SYMPATHETIC NERVOUS SYSTEM DIVISION—PARASYMPATHETIC NERVOUS SYSTEM DIVISION

Select the best answer.

83. Dendrites and cell bodies of sympathetic preganglionic neurons are located in the:
    a. Brainstem and sacral portion of the spinal cord
    b. Sympathetic ganglia
    c. Gray matter of the thoracic and upper lumbar segments of the spinal cord
    d. Ganglia close to effectors

84. Which of the following statements is *not* correct?
    a. Sympathetic preganglionic neurons have their cell bodies located in the lateral gray column of certain parts of the spinal cord.
    b. Sympathetic preganglionic axons pass along the dorsal root of certain spinal nerves.
    c. There are synapses within sympathetic ganglia.
    d. Sympathetic responses are usually widespread, involving many organs.

85. Another name for the parasympathetic nervous system is:
    a. Thoracolumbar
    b. Craniosacral
    c. Visceral
    d. ANS
    e. Cholinergic

86. Which of the following statements is *not* correct?
    a. Sympathetic postganglionic neurons have their dendrites and cell bodies in sympathetic ganglia or collateral ganglia.
    b. Sympathetic ganglions are located in front of and at each side of the spinal column.
    c. Separate autonomic nerves distribute many sympathetic postganglionic axons to various internal organs.
    d. Very few sympathetic preganglionic axons synapse with postganglionic neurons.

87. Sympathetic stimulation usually results in:
    a. Response by numerous organs
    b. Response by only one organ
    c. Increased peristalsis
    d. Constriction of pupils

88. Parasympathetic stimulation frequently results in:
    a. Response by only one organ
    b. Responses by numerous organs
    c. The "fight-or-flight" response
    d. Increased heartbeat

Select the correct term from the choices given and write the letter in the answer blank.

a. Sympathetic control
b. Parasympathetic control

89. _____ Constricts pupils

90. _____ Produces "goose pimples"

91. _____ Increases sweat secretion

92. _____ Increases secretion of digestive juices

93. _____ Constricts blood vessels

94. _____ Slows heartbeat

95. _____ Relaxes bladder

96. _____ Increases epinephrine secretion

97. _____ Increases peristalsis

98. _____ Stimulates lens for near vision

 If you had difficulty with this section, review pages 199-202.

AUTONOMIC NEUROTRANSMITTERS—AUTONOMIC NERVOUS SYSTEM AS A WHOLE

Fill in the blanks.

99. Sympathetic preganglionic axons release the neurotransmitter _____.

100. Axons that release norepinephrine are classified as _____ _____.

101. Axons that release acetylcholine are classified as _____ _____.

102. The function of the autonomic nervous system is to regulate the body's involuntary functions in ways that maintain or restore _____.

103. Your _____ _____ is determined by the combined forces of the sympathetic and parasympathetic nervous system.

104. According to some physiologists, meditation leads to _____ sympathetic activity and changes opposite to those of the "fight-or-flight" response.

 If you had difficulty with this section, review pages 202-204.

UNSCRAMBLE THE WORDS

Unscramble the circled letters and fill in the statement.

105. **R O N N E S U**

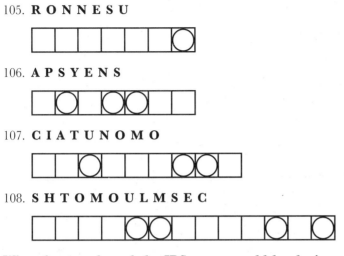

106. **A P S Y E N S**

107. **C I A T U N O M O**

108. **S H T O M O U L M S E C**

What the man hoped the IRS agent would be during his audit.

109.

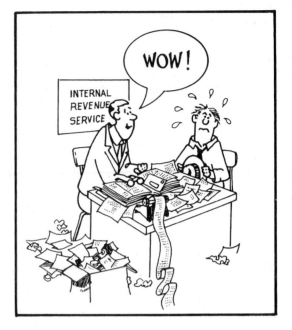

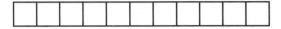

APPLYING WHAT YOU KNOW

110. Mr. Hemstreet suffered a cerebrovascular accident, and it was determined that the damage affected the left side of his cerebrum. On which side of his body will he most likely notice any paralysis?

111. Baby Dania was born with an excessive accumulation of cerebrospinal fluid in the ventricles. A catheter was placed in the ventricle and the fluid was drained by means of a shunt into the circulatory bloodstream. Which condition does this medical history describe?

112. Mrs. Muhlenkamp looked out her window to see a man trapped under the wheel of a car. Although slightly built, Mrs. Muhlenkamp rushed to the car, lifted it, and saved the man underneath the wheel. What division of the autonomic nervous system made this seemingly impossible task possible?

113. Madison's heart raced and her palms became clammy as she watched the monster movie at the local theater. When the movie was over, however, she told her friends that she was not afraid at all. She appeared to be as calm as before the movie. What division of the autonomic nervous system made this possible?

114. Bill is going to his boss for his annual evaluation. He is planning to ask for a raise and hopes the evaluation will be good. Which subdivision of the autonomic nervous system will be active during this conference? Should he have a large meal before his appointment? Support your answer with facts from the chapter.

115. WORD FIND

Can you find the 14 terms from this chapter in the box of letters? Words may be spelled top to bottom, bottom to top, right to left, left to right, or diagonally.

```
M  C  C  D  Q  S  Y  N  A  P  S  E  Q  G  O
E  N  A  Q  D  W  H  N  W  E  J  N  A  L  W
S  R  O  T  P  E  C  E  R  Y  Z  N  I  S  M
I  D  S  X  E  K  N  O  K  X  G  G  C  Y  Y
J  O  T  R  A  C  T  D  F  L  O  N  E  N  A
R  P  W  E  K  O  H  X  I  D  A  L  H  A  M
F  A  L  O  N  A  Y  O  E  I  I  I  X  P  C
C  M  Z  I  F  D  N  N  L  N  G  Z  U  T  Z
S  I  N  V  C  G  D  G  Z  A  N  A  K  I  P
G  N  A  T  Z  R  O  W  V  A  M  Y  T  C  O
K  E  N  D  O  R  P  H  I  N  S  I  L  C  X
C  P  Q  G  C  J  X  F  J  D  Q  S  N  L  F
X  U  L  I  H  I  G  Q  A  N  S  W  O  E  U
A  I  M  H  Q  E  X  K  D  B  W  Y  T  F  S
A  A  D  A  X  O  C  K  G  B  F  H  B  T  K
```

Axon	Glia	Serotonin
Catecholamines	Microglia	Synapse
Dopamine	Myelin	Synaptic cleft
Endorphins	Oligodendroglia	Tract
Ganglion	Receptors	

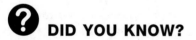

DID YOU KNOW?

- Although all pain is felt and interpreted in the brain, it has no pain sensation itself—even when cut!
- In the adult human body, there are 46 miles of nerves.
- The areas of the brain that track emotion and memory are larger and more sensitive in the female brain.
- "Rejection" actually hurts like physical pain because it triggers the same circuits in the brain.

THE NERVOUS SYSTEM

Fill in the crossword puzzle.

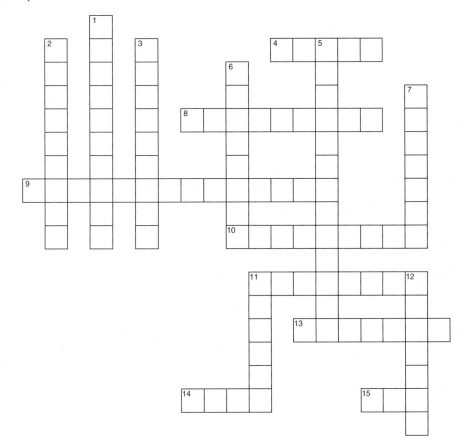

ACROSS
4. Bundle of axons located within the CNS
8. Transmits impulses toward the cell body
9. Neurons that conduct impulses from a ganglion
10. Astrocytes
11. Pia mater
13. Nerve cells
14. Transmits impulses away from the cell body
15. Peripheral nervous system (abbreviation)

DOWN
1. Neuroglia
2. Peripheral beginning of a sensory neuron's dendrite
3. Two-neuron arc (two words)
5. Neurotransmitter
6. Cluster of nerve cell bodies outside the central nervous system
7. Area of brain stem
11. Fatty substance found around some nerve fibers
12. Where impulses are transmitted from one neuron to another

CHECK YOUR KNOWLEDGE

Multiple Choice

Select the best answer.

1. Which of the following conduct impulses toward the cell body?
   a. Axons
   b. Astrocytes
   c. Microglia
   d. Dendrites

2. The outer cell membrane of a Schwann cell is called the:
   a. Glioma
   b. Neurilemma
   c. Cell body
   d. Dendrite

3. The myelin sheath in the brain and spinal cord is produced by the:
   a. Oligodendrocytes
   b. Schwann cells
   c. Microglia
   d. Blood-brain barrier

4. The simplest kind of reflex arc is a(n):
   a. One-neuron arc
   b. Two-neuron arc
   c. Three-neuron arc
   d. Action potential

5. A ganglion is a group of nerve cell bodies located in the:
   a. PNS
   b. CNS
   c. Brain and spinal cord
   d. All of the above

6. Each synaptic knob vesicle contains a very small quantity of a chemical compound called a(n):
   a. Synapse
   b. ADH
   c. Releasing hormone
   d. Neurotransmitter

7. Which of the following is located in the brainstem?
   a. Medulla oblongata
   b. Pons
   c. Midbrain
   d. All of the above

8. Which of the following is a function of the hypothalamus?
   a. Muscle coordination
   b. Willed movements
   c. Regulation of body temperature
   d. Relay for visual impulses

9. Which of the following is *not* true regarding the meninges?
   a. The tough outer layer is the dura mater.
   b. The arachnoid mater is the membrane between the dura mater and the pia mater.
   c. The pia mater resembles a "cobweb," and the name comes from the Greek word for spider.
   d. All of the above statements are true.

10. The autonomic nervous system consists of certain motor neurons that conduct impulses from the spinal cord or brainstem to the:
    a. Cardiac muscle tissue
    b. Smooth muscle tissue
    c. Glandular epithelial tissue
    d. All of the above

Matching

Select the most correct answer from column B for each statement in column A. (Only one answer is correct.)

Column A

11. _____ Multiple sclerosis

12. _____ Cerebrum

13. _____ CVA

14. _____ Cerebrospinal fluid

15. _____ Cranial nerves

16. _____ Spinal nerves

17. _____ Autonomic neurons

18. _____ Sympathetic nervous system

19. _____ Parasympathetic nervous system

20. _____ Dopamine

Column B

a. Corpus callosum
b. Abducens
c. Myelin disorder
d. Slows heartbeat
e. "Fight or flight"
f. Visceral effectors
g. Parkinson's disease
h. Ventricles
i. 31 pairs
j. Stroke

NEURONS

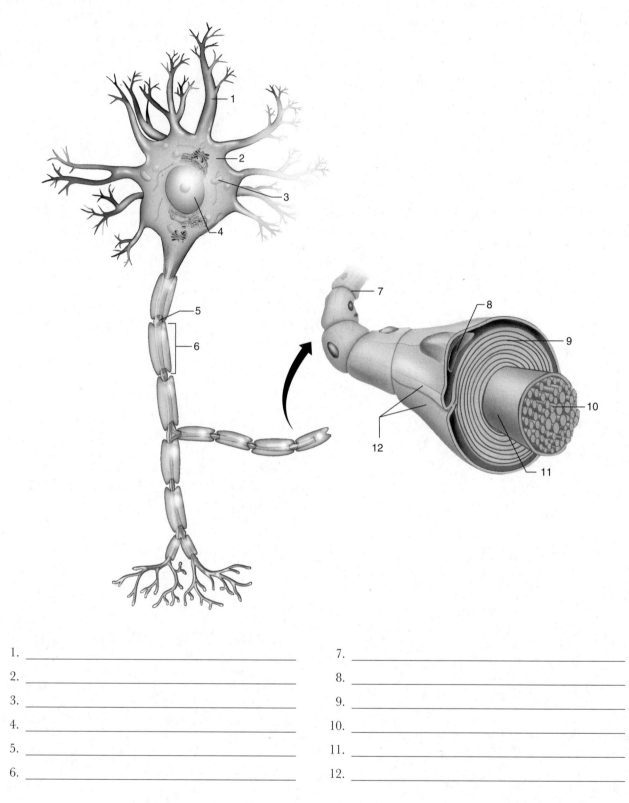

1. _____
2. _____
3. _____
4. _____
5. _____
6. _____

7. _____
8. _____
9. _____
10. _____
11. _____
12. _____

CRANIAL NERVES

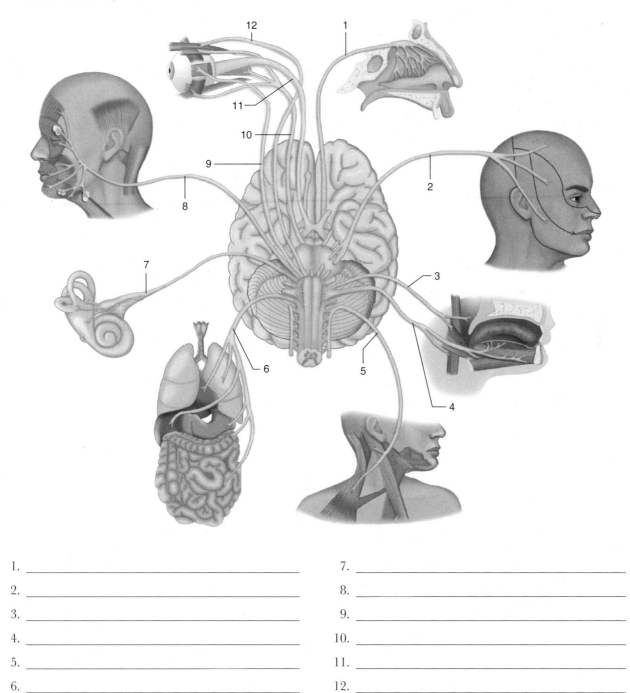

1. _____
2. _____
3. _____
4. _____
5. _____
6. _____

7. _____
8. _____
9. _____
10. _____
11. _____
12. _____

NEURAL PATHWAY INVOLVED IN THE PATELLAR REFLEX

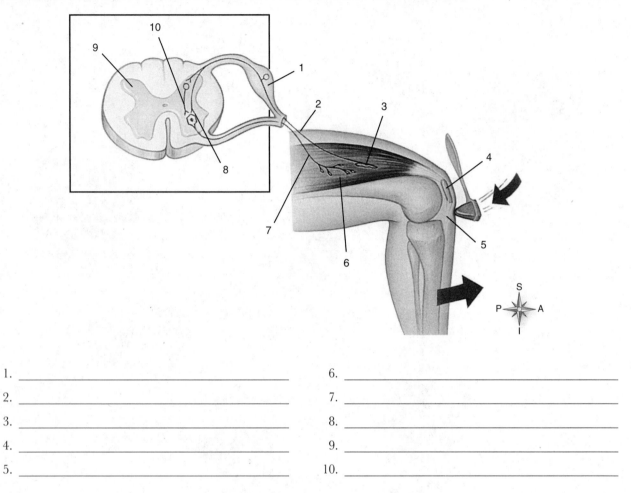

1. _____

2. _____

3. _____

4. _____

5. _____

6. _____

7. _____

8. _____

9. _____

10. _____

THE CEREBRUM

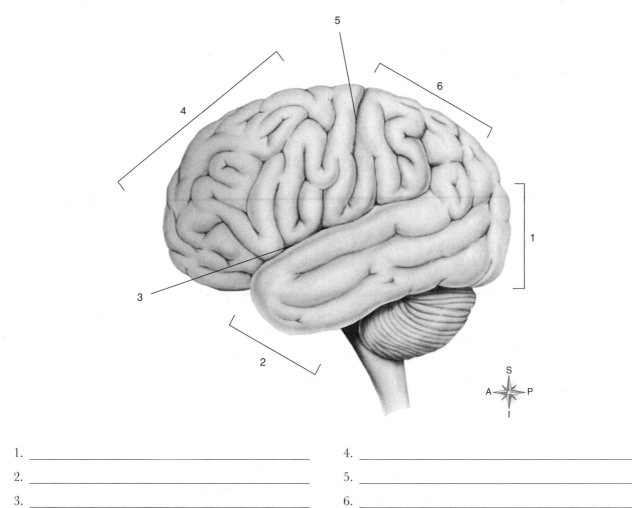

1. _____   4. _____
2. _____   5. _____
3. _____   6. _____

SAGITTAL SECTION OF THE CENTRAL NERVOUS SYSTEM

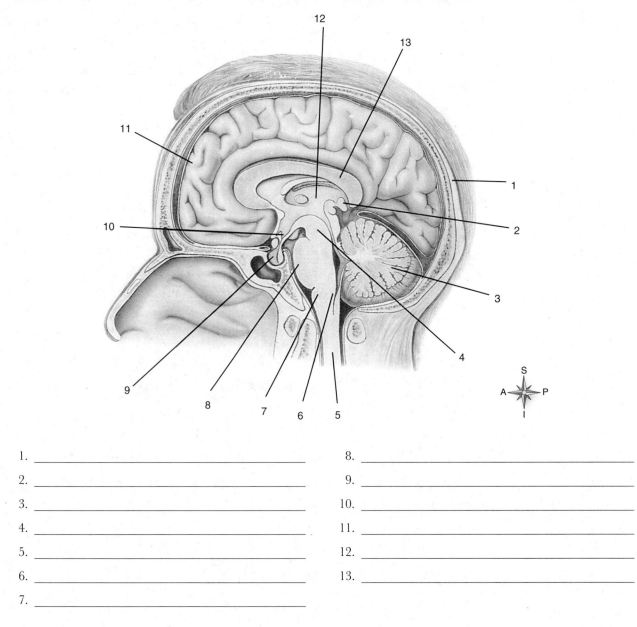

1. _____

2. _____

3. _____

4. _____

5. _____

6. _____

7. _____

8. _____

9. _____

10. _____

11. _____

12. _____

13. _____

AUTONOMIC CONDUCTION PATHS

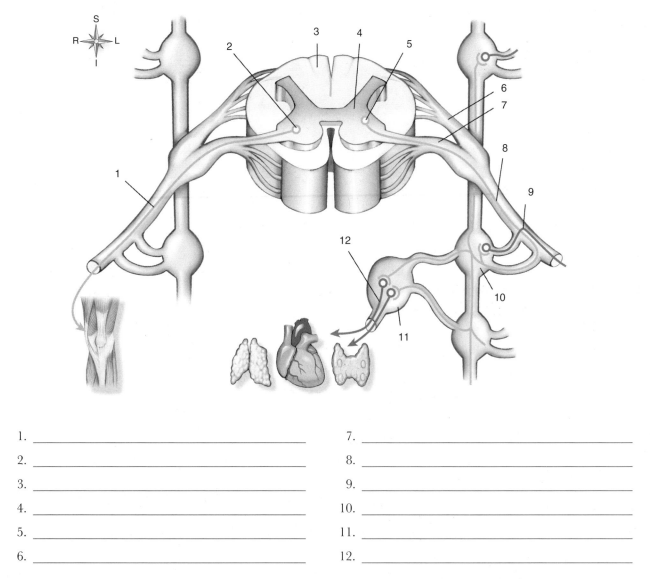

1. _____

2. _____

3. _____

4. _____

5. _____

6. _____

7. _____

8. _____

9. _____

10. _____

11. _____

12. _____

CHAPTER 10

Senses

Consider this scene for a moment. You are walking along a beautiful beach watching the sunset. You notice the various hues and are amazed at the multitude of shades that cover the sky. The waves are indeed melodious as they splash along the shore, and you wiggle your feet with delight as you sense the warm, soft sand trickling between your toes. You sip on a soda and then inhale the fresh salt air as you continue your stroll along the shore. It is a memorable scene, but one that would not be possible without the assistance of your sense organs. The sense organs pick up messages that are sent over nerve pathways to specialized areas in the brain for interpretation. They make communication with and enjoyment of the environment possible. The visual, auditory, tactile, olfactory, and gustatory sense organs not only protect us from danger but also add an important dimension to our daily pleasures of life.

Your study of this chapter will give you an understanding of another of the systems necessary for homeostasis and survival.

TOPICS FOR REVIEW

Before progressing to Chapter 11, you should review the classification of sense organs and the process for converting a stimulus into a sensation. Your study should also include an understanding of the special sense organs and the general sense organs.

SENSES—SENSORY PATHWAYS

Match the term on the left with the proper selection on the right.

Group A

1. _____ Special sense organ
2. _____ General sense organ
3. _____ Nose
4. _____ Krause's end bulbs
5. _____ Taste buds

a. Olfactory cells
b. Meissner's corpuscles
c. Chemoreceptor
d. Eye
e. Touch

Group B

6. _____ Proprioceptors
7. _____ Golgi tendon organ
8. _____ Referred pain
9. _____ Chemoreceptors
10. _____ Meissner's corpuscle

a. Detect changes in pH and CO_2 levels in the blood
b. Light touch
c. Encapsulated nerve ending
d. General sensory receptors found deep within skeletal muscle tissue
e. Stimulation of receptors in deep structures that may affect sensation far removed from site of injury or disease

→ *If you had difficulty with this section, review pages 213-216.*

SPECIAL SENSES—VISION

Multiple Choice

Select the best answer.

11. The "white" of the eye is more commonly called the:
    a. Choroid
    b. Cornea
    c. Sclera
    d. Retina
    e. None of the above

12. The "colored" part of the eye is known as the:
    a. Retina
    b. Cornea
    c. Pupil
    d. Sclera
    e. Iris

13. The transparent portion of the sclera, referred to as the *window* of the eye, is the:
    a. Retina
    b. Cornea
    c. Pupil
    d. Iris

14. The mucous membrane that covers the front of the eye is called the:
    a. Cornea
    b. Choroid
    c. Conjunctiva
    d. Ciliary body
    e. None of the above

15. The structure that can contract or dilate to allow more or less light to enter the eye is the:
    a. Lens
    b. Choroid
    c. Retina
    d. Cornea
    e. Iris

16. When the eye is looking at objects far in the distance, the lens is _____ and the ciliary muscle is _____.
    a. Rounded; contracted
    b. Rounded; relaxed
    c. Slightly rounded; contracted
    d. Slightly curved; relaxed
    e. None of the above

17. The lens of the eye is held in place by the:
    a. Ciliary muscle
    b. Aqueous humor
    c. Vitreous humor
    d. Cornea

18. When the lens loses its elasticity and can no longer bring near objects into focus, the condition is known as:
    a. Glaucoma
    b. Presbyopia
    c. Astigmatism
    d. Strabismus

19. The fluid in front of the lens that is constantly being formed, drained, and replaced in the anterior chamber is the:
    a. Vitreous humor
    b. Protoplasm
    c. Aqueous humor
    d. Conjunctiva

20. If drainage of the aqueous humor is blocked, the internal pressure within the eye will increase, and a condition known as _____ could occur.
    a. Presbyopia
    b. Glaucoma
    c. Color blindness
    d. Cataracts

21. The rods and cones are the photoreceptor cells and are located on the:
    a. Sclera
    b. Cornea
    c. Choroid
    d. Retina

22. The area that contains the greatest concentration of cones on the retina is the:
    a. Fovea centralis
    b. Retinal artery
    c. Ciliary body
    d. Optic disc

23. If our eyes are abnormally elongated, the image focuses in front of the retina, and a condition known as _____ occurs.
    a. Hyperopia
    b. Cataracts
    c. Night blindness
    d. Myopia

➡ *If you had difficulty with this section, review pages 216-221.*

HEARING AND EQUILIBRIUM

Select the correct term from the choices given and write the letter in the answer blank.

a. External ear
b. Middle ear
c. Inner ear

24. _____ Malleus

25. _____ Perilymph

26. _____ Incus

27. _____ Ceruminous glands

28. _____ Cochlea

29. _____ Acoustic canal

30. _____ Semicircular canals

31. _____ Stapes

32. _____ Eustachian tube

33. _____ Organ of Corti

Fill in the blanks.

34. The external ear has two parts: the _____ and the _____

    _____ _____.

35. Another name for the tympanic membrane is the _____.

36. The bones of the middle ear are collectively referred to as _____.

37. The stapes presses against a membrane that covers a small opening called the _____

    _____.

38. A middle ear infection is called _____ _____.

39. The _____ is located adjacent to the oval window between the semicircular canals and the cochlea.

40. Located within the semicircular canals and the vestibule are _____ for balance and equilibrium.

41. The sensory cells in the _____ _____ are stimulated when movement of the head causes the endolymph to move.

➡ *If you had difficulty with this section, review pages 222-226.*

TASTE AND SMELL

Circle the correct answer.

42. Structures known as (*papillae* or *olfactory cells*) are found on the tongue.

43. Nerve impulses generated by stimulation of taste buds travel primarily through two (*cranial* or *spinal*) nerves.

44. To be detected by olfactory receptors, chemicals must be dissolved in the watery (*mucus* or *plasma*) that lines the nasal cavity.

45. The pathways taken by olfactory nerve impulses and the areas where these impulses are interpreted are closely associated with areas of the brain important in (*hearing* or *memory*).

46. (*Chemoreceptor* or *Mechanoreceptor*) is the term used to describe the types of receptors that generate nervous impulses resulting in the sense of taste or smell.

➡ *If you had difficulty with this section, review pages 226-229.*

UNSCRAMBLE THE WORDS

Unscramble the circled letters and fill in the statement.

47. **C A L R I E U**

□ ⓞ □ □ □ □ □

48. **R A E C L S**

ⓞ □ ⓞ □ □ □

49. **L A P I L A E P**

ⓞ □ ⓞ □ □ □ □ □

50. **C T V N U C N O I A J**

□ □ □ □ □ □ □ ⓞ □ □

What Mr. Tuttle liked best about his classroom.

51.

□ □ □ □ □ □ □

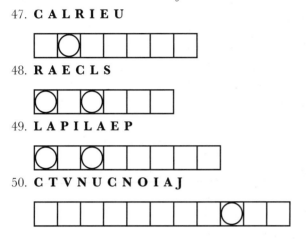

 APPLYING WHAT YOU KNOW

52. Mr. Nay was an avid swimmer and competed regularly in his age group. He had to withdraw from the last competition due to an infection of his ear. Antibiotics and analgesics were prescribed by the doctor. What is the medical term for his condition?

53. Mrs. Metheny loved the outdoors and spent a great deal of her spare time basking in the sun on the beach. Her physician suggested that she begin wearing sunglasses regularly when he noticed milky spots beginning to appear on Mrs. Metheny's lenses. What condition was Mrs. Metheny's physician trying to prevent?

54. Shelley repeatedly became ill with throat infections during her first few years of school. Lately, however, she has noticed that whenever she has a throat infection, her ears become very sore also. What might be the cause of this additional problem?

55. Julius was hit in the nose with a baseball during practice. His sense of smell was temporarily gone. Which nerve receptors were damaged during the injury?

56. WORD FIND

Can you find the 19 terms from this chapter in the box of letters? Words may be spelled top to bottom, bottom to top, right to left, left to right, or diagonally.

```
M E C H A N O R E C E P T O R
H R A T B Q I R T B N H M A E
P F T Y R O T C A F L O X R C
G U A Y I N A I H C A T S U E
G P R A C E R U M E N O P X P
I E A I P O Y B S E R P K D T
W L C P L Y N E Y K E I T O O
C Q T O I B R J B S F G L M R
Z U S R C L E O U J R M N N S
F D M E O H L Q T N A E Y I S
H I D P N D L A M A C N X S Z
A M L Y E S S E E D T T M Z H
D D M H S F E X A Y I S I I A
J C G N J T I S L P O G U V J
P H G Y A K H S U C N I S G A
```

Cataracts	Gustatory	Presbyopia
Cerumen	Hyperopia	Receptors
Cochlea	Incus	Refraction
Cones	Mechanoreceptor	Rods
Conjunctiva	Olfactory	Senses
Eustachian	Papillae	
Eye	Photopigment	

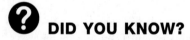 **DID YOU KNOW?**

- The human eye blinks an average of 4,200,000 times a year.
- Our eyes are always the same size from birth, but our nose and ears never stop growing.
- If your mouth was completely dry, you would not be able to distinguish the taste of anything.
- Tongue prints are as unique as fingerprints.

THE SENSES

Fill in the crossword puzzle.

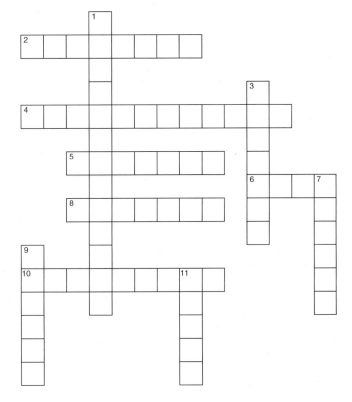

ACROSS
2. Bones of the middle ear
4. Located in anterior cavity in front of lens (two words)
5. External ear
6. Transparent body behind pupil
8. Front part of this coat is the ciliary muscle and iris
10. Membranous labyrinth filled with this fluid

DOWN
1. Located in posterior cavity (two words)
3. Organ of Corti located here
7. White of the eye
9. Innermost layer of the eye
11. Hole in center of the iris

CHECK YOUR KNOWLEDGE

Multiple Choice

Select the best answer.

1. The Golgi tendon receptors and muscle spindles are important:
   a. Proprioceptors
   b. Photoreceptors
   c. Chemoreceptors
   d. None of the above

2. Another name for *farsightedness* is:
   a. Myopia
   b. Hyperopia
   c. Astigmatism
   d. None of the above

3. In addition to its role in hearing, the ear also functions as:
   a. The sense organ of equilibrium and balance
   b. A sense organ for chemoreceptors
   c. The sense organ for gustatory cells
   d. None of the above

4. The occipital lobe is responsible for:
   a. Interpretation of mechanoreceptors
   b. Interpretation of chemoreceptors
   c. Visual interpretation
   d. None of the above

5. Another name for the tympanic membrane is the:
   a. Ossicle
   b. Eardrum
   c. External auditory canal
   d. Oval window

6. The inner ear consists of three spaces in the temporal bone, assembled in a complex maze called the:
   a. Crista ampullaris
   b. Bony labyrinth
   c. Organ of Corti
   d. Ossicles

7. Three layers of tissue form the eyeball. They are the:
   a. Iris, conjunctiva, and cornea
   b. Choroid, iris, and pupil
   c. Retina, rods, and cones
   d. Fibrous, vascular, and inner layer

8. The jellylike fluid behind the lens in the posterior chamber is the:
   a. Aqueous humor
   b. Vitreous humor
   c. Endolymph
   d. Perilymph

9. The eustachian tube connects the throat with the:
   a. Tympanic membrane
   b. External ear
   c. Inner ear
   d. Middle ear

10. The receptors for night vision are the:
    a. Rods
    b. Cones
    c. Fovea centralis
    d. Chemoreceptors

True or False

If the statement is true, write "T" in the answer blank. If the statement is false, correct the statement by circling the incorrect term and writing the correct term in the answer blank.

11. _____ The sense organs are often classified as either general sense organs or special sense organs.

12. _____ The cornea is sometimes spoken of as the *white of the eye.*

13. _____ Several involuntary muscles make up the front part of the choroid.

14. _____ When the lens becomes hard and loses its transparency, a condition called *glaucoma* occurs.

15. _____ The organ of Corti is also known as the *organ of hearing.*

16. _____ The optic disc is also known as the *blind spot.*

17. _____ The malleus, incus, and stapes are also known as the *ossicles.*

18. _____ A middle ear infection may also be referred to as *otitis media.*

19. _____ The chemoreceptors of the taste buds are called *gustatory cells.*

20. _____ Tears are formed in the lacrimal gland.

EYE

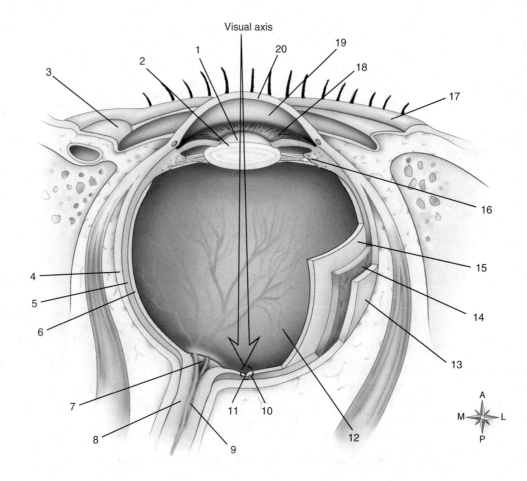

Visual axis

1. _____
2. _____
3. _____
4. _____
5. _____
6. _____
7. _____
8. _____
9. _____
10. _____

11. _____
12. _____
13. _____
14. _____
15. _____
16. _____
17. _____
18. _____
19. _____
20. _____

EAR

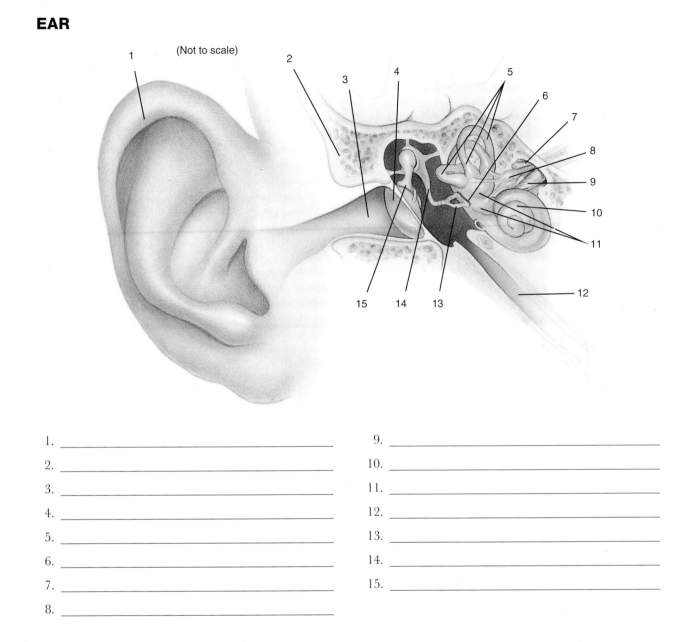

(Not to scale)

1. _____

2. _____

3. _____

4. _____

5. _____

6. _____

7. _____

8. _____

9. _____

10. _____

11. _____

12. _____

13. _____

14. _____

15. _____

Endocrine System

The endocrine system has often been compared to a fine symphony concert. When all instruments are playing properly, the sound is melodious. If one instrument plays too loudly or too softly, however, it affects the overall quality of the performance.

The endocrine system is a ductless system that releases hormones into the bloodstream to help regulate body functions. The pituitary gland may be considered the conductor of the orchestra, as it stimulates many of the endocrine glands to secrete their powerful hormones. All hormones, whether stimulated in this manner or by other control mechanisms, are interdependent. A change in the level of one hormone may affect the level and performance of many other hormones.

In addition to the endocrine glands, prostaglandins ("tissue hormones") are powerful substances similar to hormones that have been found in a variety of body tissues. These hormones are often produced in a tissue and diffuse only a short distance to act on cells within that area. Prostaglandins influence respiration, blood pressure, gastrointestinal secretions, and the reproductive system, and they may someday play an important role in the treatment of diseases such as hypertension, asthma, and ulcers.

The endocrine system is a system of communication and control. It differs from the nervous system in that hormones provide a slower, longer-lasting effect than do nerve stimuli and responses. Your understanding of the "system of hormones" will alert you to the mechanism of our emotions; responses to stress, growth, chemical balances; and many other body functions.

TOPICS FOR REVIEW

Before progressing to Chapter 12, you should be able to identify and locate the primary endocrine glands of the body. Your understanding should include the hormones that are produced by these glands and the method by which these secretions are regulated. Your study will conclude with the pathological conditions that result from the malfunctioning of this system.

ENDOCRINE GLANDS—MECHANISMS OF HORMONE ACTION—REGULATION OF HORMONE SECRETION—PROSTAGLANDINS

Match the term on the left with the proper selection on the right.

Group A

1. _____ Pituitary	a. Pelvic cavity	
2. _____ Parathyroids	b. Mediastinum	
	c. Neck	
3. _____ Adrenals	d. Cranial cavity	
4. _____ Ovaries	e. Abdominal cavity	
5. _____ Thymus		

Group B

6. _____ Negative feedback	a. Cyclic AMP is an example of one
7. _____ Tissue hormones	b. Respond to a particular hormone
	c. Prostaglandins
8. _____ Second messenger	d. Discharge secretions into ducts
9. _____ Exocrine glands	e. Specialized homeostatic mechanism that regulates release of hormones
10. _____ Target organ cells	

Fill in the blanks.

Nonsteroid hormones serve as (11) _____ _____ providing communication between (12) _____ and (13) _____ _____. Another molecule such as (14) _____ _____ then acts as the (15) _____ _____ providing (16) _____ within a hormone's (17) _____ _____.

➡ *If you had difficulty with this section, review pages 237-242.*

PITUITARY GLAND—HYPOTHALAMUS

Select the best answer.

18. The pituitary gland lies in the _____ bone.
    a. Ethmoid
    b. Sphenoid
    c. Temporal
    d. Frontal
    e. Occipital

19. Which one of the following structures would *not* be stimulated by a tropic hormone from the anterior pituitary?
    a. Ovaries
    b. Testes
    c. Thyroid
    d. Adrenals
    e. Uterus

20. Which one of the following is *not* a function of FSH?
    a. Stimulates the growth of follicles
    b. Stimulates the production of estrogens
    c. Stimulates the growth of seminiferous tubules
    d. Stimulates the interstitial cells of the testes

21. Which one of the following is *not* a function of LH?
    a. Stimulates maturation of a developing follicle
    b. Stimulates the production of estrogens
    c. Stimulates the formation of a corpus luteum
    d. Stimulates sperm cells to mature in the male
    e. Causes ovulation

22. Which one of the following is *not* a function of GH?
    a. Increases glucose catabolism
    b. Increases fat catabolism
    c. Speeds up the movement of amino acids into cells from the bloodstream
    d. All of the above are functions of GH

23. Which one of the following hormones is *not* released by the anterior pituitary gland?
    a. ACTH
    b. TSH
    c. ADH
    d. FSH
    e. LH

24. Which one of the following is *not* a function of prolactin?
    a. Stimulates breast development during pregnancy
    b. Stimulates milk secretion after delivery
    c. Causes the release of milk from glandular cells of the breast
    d. All of the above are functions of prolactin

25. The anterior pituitary gland secretes:
    a. Eight major hormones
    b. Tropic hormones that stimulate other endocrine glands to grow and secrete
    c. ADH
    d. Oxytocin

26. TSH acts on the:
    a. Thyroid
    b. Thymus
    c. Pineal
    d. Testes

27. ACTH stimulates the:
    a. Adrenal cortex
    b. Adrenal medulla
    c. Hypothalamus
    d. Ovaries

28. Which hormone is secreted by the posterior pituitary gland?
    a. MSH
    b. LH
    c. GH
    d. ADH

29. ADH serves the body by:
    a. Initiating labor
    b. Accelerating water reabsorption from urine into the blood
    c. Stimulating the pineal gland
    d. Regulating the calcium/phosphorus levels in the blood

30. Which disease is caused by hyposecretion of ADH?
    a. Diabetes insipidus
    b. Diabetes mellitus
    c. Acromegaly
    d. Myxedema

31. The actual production of ADH and oxytocin takes place in the:
    a. Anterior pituitary
    b. Posterior pituitary
    c. Hypothalamus
    d. Pineal

32. Inhibiting hormones are produced by the:
    a. Anterior pituitary
    b. Posterior pituitary
    c. Hypothalamus
    d. Pineal

Select the correct term from the choices given and write the letter in the answer blank.

a. Anterior pituitary
b. Posterior pituitary
c. Hypothalamus

33. _____ Adenohypophysis

34. _____ Neurohypophysis

35. _____ Induced labor

36. _____ Appetite

37. _____ Acromegaly

38. _____ Body temperature

39. _____ Sex hormones

40. _____ Tropic hormones

41. _____ Gigantism

42. _____ Releasing hormones

➜ *If you had difficulty with this section, review pages 242-245.*

THYROID GLAND—PARATHYROID GLANDS

Circle the correct answer.

43. The thyroid gland lies (*above* or *below*) the larynx.

44. The thyroid gland secretes (*calcitonin* or *glucagon*).

45. For thyroxine to be produced in adequate amounts, the diet must contain sufficient (*calcium* or *iodine*).

46. Most endocrine glands (*do* or *do not*) store their hormones.

47. Colloid is a storage medium for the (*thyroid* or *parathyroid*) hormone.

48. Calcitonin (*increases* or *decreases*) the concentration of calcium in the blood.

49. Simple goiter results from (*hyperthyroidism* or *hypothyroidism*).

50. Hyposecretion of thyroid hormones during the formative years leads to (*cretinism* or *myxedema*).

51. The parathyroid glands secrete the hormone (*PTH* or *PTA*).

52. Parathyroid hormone tends to (*increase* or *decrease*) the concentration of calcium in the blood.

➜ *If you had difficulty with this section, review pages 245-247.*

ADRENAL GLANDS

Fill in the blanks.

53. The adrenal gland is actually two separate endocrine glands: the _____ _____ and the _____ _____.

54. Hormones secreted by the adrenal cortex are known as _____.

55. The outer zone of the adrenal cortex secretes _____.

56. The middle zone secretes _____.

57. The innermost zone secretes _____ _____.

58. Glucocorticoids act in several ways to increase _____.

59. Glucocorticoids also play an essential part in maintaining _____ _____.

60. The adrenal medulla secretes the hormones _____ and _____.

61. The adrenal medulla may help the body resist _____.

62. Deficiency or hyposecretion of adrenal cortex hormones results in a condition called _____ _____.

Select the correct term from the choices given and write the letter in the answer blank.

a. Adrenal cortex
b. Adrenal medulla

63. _____ Mineralocorticoids

64. _____ Anti-immunity

65. _____ Adrenaline

66. _____ Cushing syndrome

67. _____ "Fight-or-flight" response

68. _____ Aldosterone

69. _____ Androgens

➡ *If you had difficulty with this section, review pages 247-250.*

PANCREATIC ISLETS, SEX GLANDS, THYMUS, PLACENTA, PINEAL GLAND

Circle the term that does not *belong.*

70. Alpha cells	Glucagon	Beta cells	Glycogenolysis
71. Insulin	Glucagon	Beta cells	Diabetes mellitus
72. Estrogens	Progesterone	Corpus luteum	Thymosin
73. Chorion	Interstitial cells	Testosterone	Semen
74. Immune system	Mediastinum	Aldosterone	Thymosin
75. Pregnancy	ACTH	Estrogen	Chorion
76. Melatonin	Menstruation	"Third eye"	Semen

Match the term on the left with the proper selection on the right.

Group A

77. _____ Alpha cells
78. _____ Beta cells
79. _____ Corpus luteum
80. _____ Interstitial cells
81. _____ Ovarian follicles

a. Estrogen
b. Progesterone
c. Insulin
d. Testosterone
e. Glucagon

Group B

82. _____ Placenta
83. _____ Pineal
84. _____ Heart atria
85. _____ Testes
86. _____ Thymus

a. Melatonin
b. ANH
c. Testosterone
d. Thymosin
e. Chorionic gonadotropins

➡ *If you had difficulty with this section, review pages 250-253.*

ENDOCRINE FUNCTIONS THROUGHOUT THE BODY

True or False

If the statement is true, write "T" in the answer blank. If the statement is false, correct the statement by circling the incorrect term and writing the correct term in the answer blank.

87. _____ Almost every organ and system has an endocrine function.

88. _____ ANH is an antagonist to aldosterone.

89. _____ Ghrelin regulates how hungry or full we feel and how the body metabolizes fat.

90. _____ Aldosterone stimulates the kidney to retain sodium ions and water, and ANH stimulates loss of sodium ions and water.

91. _____ Leptin is secreted by epithelial cells lining the stomach and boosts appetite, slows metabolism, and reduces fat burning.

➡ *If you had difficulty with this section, review pages 253-255.*

UNSCRAMBLE THE WORDS

Unscramble the circled letters and fill in the statement.

92. **R O O D I I T S C C**

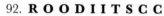

93. **S I U I S E R D**

94. **U O O O T D C S I I L R C C G**

95. **R I O D S T E S**

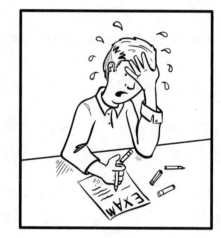

Why Billy didn't like to take exams.

96.

APPLYING WHAT YOU KNOW

97. Mrs. Langston made a routine visit to her physician last week. When the laboratory results came back, the report indicated a high level of chorionic gonadotropin in her urine. What did this mean to Mrs. Langston?

98. Mrs. Wilcox noticed that her daughter was beginning to take on some of the secondary sex characteristics of a male. The pediatrician diagnosed the condition as a tumor of an endocrine gland. Where specifically was the tumor located?

99. Mrs. Florez was pregnant and was 2 weeks past her due date. Her doctor suggested that she enter the hospital and said he would induce labor. Which hormone will he give Mrs. Florez?

100. WORD FIND

Can you find the 16 terms from the chapter in the box of letters? Words may be spelled top to bottom, bottom to top, right to left, left to right, or diagonally.

```
S S I S E R U I D M E S I T W
N D N X E B A M E D E X Y M I
I I G O N R S G X T I I Y V B
D O M S I N I T E R C C U Q D
N C X S R T N B O T V M Y O M
A I M E C L A C R E P Y H I X
L T Y R O I E Z Q R T J V K F
G R E T D P S N I L D J M X N
A O O S N I D K I N K S P P O
T C P R E T I O G R I F M X G
S L M H Y P O G L Y C E M I A
O A J L H O R M O N E O T G C
R C E L T S E L C N P N X U U
P I O S W R T X C G U L O E L
G G V Y H M S H Y K A K N Q G
```

Corticoids	Glucagon	Myxedema
Cretinism	Goiter	Prostaglandins
Diabetes	Hormone	Steroids
Diuresis	Hypercalcemia	Stress
Endocrine	Hypoglycemia	
Exocrine	Luteinization	

❓ DID YOU KNOW?

- The pituitary weighs little more than a small paper clip.
- The total daily output of the pituitary gland is less than 1/1,000,000 of a gram, yet this small amount is responsible for stimulating the majority of all endocrine functions.
- There are almost 30 hormones that are continuously being produced for us by various glands of the endocrine system.

THE ENDOCRINE SYSTEM

Fill in the crossword puzzle.

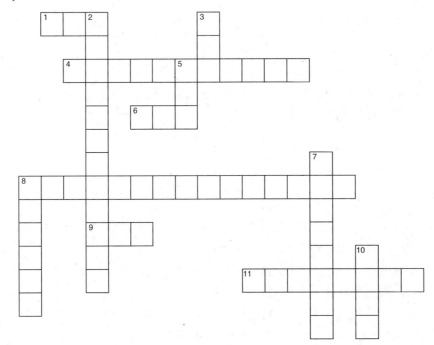

ACROSS

1. Secreted by cells in the walls of the heart's atria
4. Adrenal medulla
6. Estrogens
8. Converts amino acids to glucose
9. Melanin
11. Labor

DOWN

2. Hypersecretion of insulin
3. Antagonist to diuresis
5. Increases calcium concentration
7. Hyposecretion of islets of Langerhans (one word)
8. Hyposecretion of thyroid
10. Adrenal cortex

CHECK YOUR KNOWLEDGE

Multiple Choice

Select the best answer.

1. All of the following are included in the endocrine system *except:*
   a. Exocrine glands
   b. Steroid hormones
   c. Nonsteroid hormones
   d. All of the above are included in the endocrine system

2. The luteinizing hormone (LH) stimulates:
   a. Breast development during pregnancy
   b. The development of ovarian follicles
   c. Maturation of ovarian follicle and triggers ovulation
   d. Seminiferous tubules of testes to grow and produce sperm

3. Prostaglandins or tissue hormones influence:
   a. Respiration
   b. Gastrointestinal secretions
   c. Blood pressure
   d. All of the above

4. Which of the following is *not* stimulated by the anterior pituitary gland?
   a. TSH
   b. ACTH
   c. ADH
   d. FSH

5. Too much insulin in the blood:
   a. Has the same effect on blood glucose as the growth hormone
   b. Increases blood glucose concentration
   c. Stimulates retention of water by the kidneys
   d. Produces hypoglycemia

6. The posterior pituitary gland and hypothalamus:
   a. Release two hormones
   b. Produce substances called *releasing* and *inhibiting* hormones
   c. Cause the glandular cells of the breast to release milk into ducts for nursing a baby
   d. All of the above

7. In addition to producing thyroid hormones, the thyroid gland also secretes:
   a. Hydrocortisone
   b. Calcitonin
   c. Aldosterone
   d. Glucagon

8. The adrenal medulla produces hormones that are:
   a. Not essential for life
   b. Helpful in responding to stress
   c. Responsible for the "fight-or-flight" response
   d. All of the above

9. The pineal gland produces several hormones in small quantities, with the most significant being:
   a. ANH
   b. Leptin
   c. Chorionic gonadotropins
   d. Melatonin

10. What plays a critical role in the body's defenses against infections?
    a. Pancreas
    b. Thymus
    c. Pineal body
    d. Thyroid

Matching

Select the most correct answer from column B for each statement in column A. (Only one answer is correct.)

Column A

11. _____ Steroid hormones

12. _____ Positive feedback

13. _____ Tropic hormones

14. _____ Myxedema

15. _____ Glucocorticoids

16. _____ Aldosterone

17. _____ Islets of Langerhans

18. _____ Glycosuria

19. _____ Pineal gland

20. _____ Corpus luteum

Column B

a. Pancreas
b. Adrenal cortex
c. Progesterone
d. Diabetes mellitus
e. "Third eye"
f. Mineralocorticoid
g. Occurs during labor
h. Anterior pituitary
i. Thyroid gland
j. Lipid soluble

ENDOCRINE GLANDS

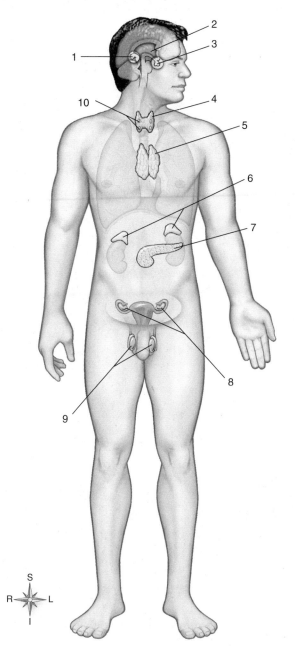

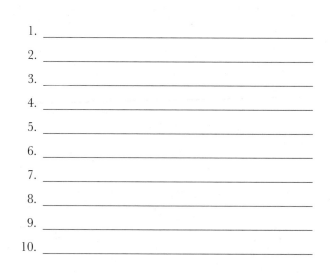

1. _____

2. _____

3. _____

4. _____

5. _____

6. _____

7. _____

8. _____

9. _____

10. _____

CHAPTER **12**

Blood

Blood, the river of life, is the body's primary means of transportation. Although it is the respiratory system that provides oxygen for the body, the digestive system that provides nutrients, and the urinary system that eliminates wastes, none of these functions could be provided for the individual cells without the blood. In less than 1 minute, a drop of blood will complete a trip through the entire body, distributing nutrients and collecting the wastes of metabolism.

Blood is divided into plasma (the liquid portion of blood) and the formed elements (the blood cells). There are three types of blood cells: red blood cells, white blood cells, and platelets. Together these cells and plasma provide a means of transportation that delivers the body's daily necessities.

Although the red blood cells in all of us are of a similar shape, we have different blood types. Blood types are identified by the presence of certain antigens in the red blood cells. Every person's blood belongs to one of four main blood groups: type A, B, AB, or O. Any one of the four groups or "types" may or may not have the specific antigen called the *Rh factor* present in the red blood cells. If an individual has the Rh factor present in his or her blood, the blood is Rh positive. If this factor is missing, the blood is Rh negative. Approximately 85% of the population has the Rh factor (Rh positive), and 15% do not have the Rh factor (Rh negative).

Your understanding of this chapter will be necessary to prepare a proper foundation for the circulatory system.

TOPICS FOR REVIEW

Before progressing to Chapter 13, you should have an understanding of the structure and function of blood plasma and cells. Your review should also include knowledge of blood types and Rh factors.

BLOOD COMPOSITION—RED BLOOD CELLS

Multiple Choice

Select the best answer.

1. Which one of the following substances is *not* a part of the plasma?
   a. Hormones
   b. Salts
   c. Nutrients
   d. Wastes
   e. All of the above are part of the plasma

2. The normal volume of blood in an adult is about:
   a. 2-3 pints
   b. 2-3 quarts
   c. 2-3 gallons
   d. 4-6 liters

3. Another name for red blood cells is:
   a. Leukocytes
   b. Thrombocytes
   c. Platelets
   d. Erythrocytes

4. Another name for white blood cells is:
   a. Erythrocytes
   b. Leukocytes
   c. Thrombocytes
   d. Platelets

5. Another name for platelets is:
   a. Neutrophils
   b. Eosinophils
   c. Thrombocytes
   d. Erythrocytes

6. Pernicious anemia is caused by:
   a. A lack of vitamin B_{12}
   b. Hemorrhage
   c. Radiation
   d. Bleeding ulcers

7. The laboratory test called *hematocrit* tells the physician the volume of:
   a. White cells in a blood sample
   b. Red cells in a blood sample
   c. Platelets in a blood sample
   d. Plasma in a blood sample

8. An example of an agranular leukocyte is a(n):
   a. Platelet
   b. Erythrocyte
   c. Eosinophil
   d. Monocyte

9. Which is *not* a formed element?
   a. Leukocytes
   b. Erythrocytes
   c. Globulins
   d. Platelets

10. A critical component of hemoglobin is:
    a. Potassium
    b. Calcium
    c. Vitamin K
    d. Iron

11. Sickle cell anemia is caused by the production of:
    a. An abnormal type of hemoglobin
    b. Excessive neutrophils
    c. Excessive platelets
    d. Abnormal leukocytes

12. The practice of using blood transfusions to increase oxygen delivery to muscles during athletic events is called blood:
    a. Antigen
    b. Doping
    c. Agglutination
    d. Proofing

13. Myeloid tissue is _____ tissue.
    a. Epithelial
    b. Connective
    c. Muscle
    d. Nervous

14. Which one of the following types of cells is *not* a granular leukocyte?
    a. Neutrophil
    b. Lymphocyte
    c. Basophil
    d. Eosinophil

15. If a blood cell has no nucleus and is shaped like a biconcave disc, then the cell most likely is a(n):
    a. Platelet
    b. Lymphocyte
    c. Basophil
    d. Eosinophil
    e. Red blood cell

16. Red bone marrow forms all kinds of blood cells *except:*
    a. Platelets
    b. Lymphocytes
    c. Red blood cells
    d. Neutrophils

17. Myeloid tissue is found in all of the following locations *except:*
    a. Sternum
    b. Ribs
    c. Wrist bones
    d. Hip bones
    e. Cranial bones

18. Lymphatic tissue is found in all of the following locations *except:*
    a. Lymph nodes
    b. Thymus
    c. Spleen
    d. All of the above contain lymphatic tissue

19. The "buffy coat" layer in a hematocrit tube contains:
    a. Red blood cells and platelets
    b. Plasma only
    c. Platelets only
    d. White blood cells and platelets
    e. None of the above

20. The hematocrit value for red blood cells should be:
    a. 75%
    b. 60%
    c. 50%
    d. 45%
    e. 35%

➡ *If you had difficulty with this section, review pages 262-269.*

BLOOD TYPES—RH FACTOR

21. *Fill in the missing areas of the chart.*

Blood Type	Antigen Present in RBCs	Antibody Present in Plasma
A		Anti-B
B	B	
AB		None
O	None	

Fill in the blanks.

22. A(n) _____ is a substance that can stimulate the body to make antibodies.

23. A(n) _____ is a substance made by the body in response to stimulation by an antigen.

24. Many antibodies react with their antigens to clump or _____ them.

25. If a baby is born to an Rh-negative mother and Rh-positive father, it may develop the disease _____ _____ .

26. The term *Rh* is used because the antigen was first discovered in the blood of a(n) _____ _____ .

27. _____ stops an Rh-negative mother from forming anti-Rh antibodies and thus prevents the possibility of harm to the next Rh-positive baby.

28. Blood type _____ has been called the *universal recipient*.

➲ *If you had difficulty with this section, review pages 269-271.*

WHITE BLOOD CELLS—PLATELETS—BLOOD CLOTTING

Multiple Choice

Select the best answer.

29. An unusually low white blood cell count would be termed:
    a. Leukemia
    b. Leukopenia
    c. Leukocytosis
    d. Anemia
    e. None of the above

30. The most numerous of the phagocytes are the _____ .
    a. Lymphocytes
    b. Neutrophils
    c. Basophils
    d. Eosinophils
    e. Monocytes

31. Which one of the following types of cells is *not* phagocytic?
    a. Neutrophils
    b. Eosinophils
    c. Lymphocytes
    d. Monocytes
    e. All of the above are phagocytic cells

32. Which of the following cell types functions in the immune process?
    a. Neutrophils
    b. Lymphocytes
    c. Monocytes
    d. Basophils
    e. Reticuloendothelial cells

33. The organ that manufactures prothrombin is the:
    a. Liver
    b. Pancreas
    c. Thymus
    d. Kidney
    e. Spleen

34. Which one of the following vitamins acts to accelerate blood clotting?
    a. A
    b. B
    c. C
    d. D
    e. K

35. Vitamin K stimulates liver cells to increase the synthesis of:
    a. Prothrombin
    b. Thrombin
    c. Platelets
    d. Heparin
    e. Calcium

36. Thrombocytes are:
    a. Tiny cell fragments
    b. Filled with chemicals necessary to initiate blood clotting
    c. Formed elements
    d. All of the above

37. If part of a clot dislodges and circulates through the bloodstream, the dislodged part is called a(n):
    a. Thrombus
    b. Thrombosis
    c. Anticoagulant
    d. Clotting factor
    e. Embolus

38. Which of the following is *not* a critical component of coagulation?
    a. Thrombin
    b. Fibrinolysis
    c. Fibrinogen
    d. Fibrin

39. Which of the following does *not* hasten clotting?
    a. A rough spot in the endothelium
    b. Abnormally slow blood flow
    c. Heparin
    d. All of the above hasten clotting

Circle the correct response.

40. Tissue plasminogen activator (TPA) is used to dissolve (*heart* or *hemorrhagic stroke*) clots.

41. An international normalized ratio (INR) of (*0.8* or *2.5*) is normal.

42. When a clot stays in the place where it formed, it is called a (*fibrin* or *thrombus*).

43. The most widely used anticoagulant is (*low-dose aspirin* or *heparin*).

44. A lab test called the PT is used to regulate the dosage of (*anticoagulant drugs* or *RhoGAM*).

45. A professional who collects blood for testing or storage is a (*phlebotomist* or *clinical laboratory technician*).

➜ *If you had difficulty with this section, review pages 271-276.*

UNSCRAMBLE THE WORDS

Unscramble the circled letters and fill in the statement.

46. **H G A P O Y C E T**

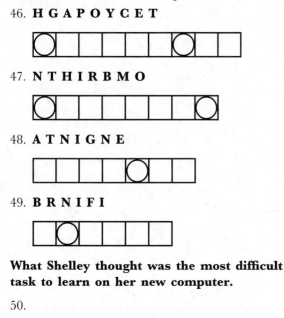

47. **N T H I R B M O**

48. **A T N I G N E**

49. **B R N I F I**

What Shelley thought was the most difficult task to learn on her new computer.

50.

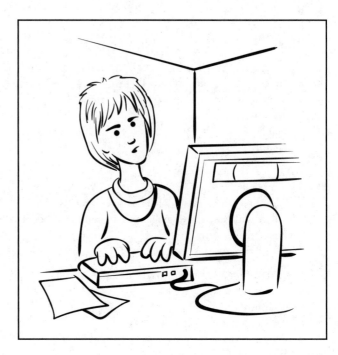

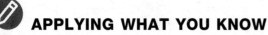

APPLYING WHAT YOU KNOW

51. Mrs. Lassiter's blood type is O positive. Her husband's type is O negative. Her newborn baby's blood type is O negative. Is there any need for concern with this combination?

52. After Mrs. Freund's baby was born, the doctor applied a gauze dressing for a short time on the umbilical cord. He also gave the baby a dose of vitamin K. Why did the doctor perform these two procedures?

53. WORD FIND

Can you find 24 terms from this chapter in the box of letters? Words may be spelled top to bottom, bottom to top, right to left, left to right, or diagonally.

```
H  S  H  K  L  S  U  L  O  B  M  E  A  E  S
K  E  E  V  M  Z  H  E  P  A  R  I  N  D  N
D  T  M  F  A  C  T  O  R  Y  E  T  I  Q  P
O  Y  A  O  H  N  B  A  T  Q  Y  A  R  A  R
N  C  T  J  G  W  E  H  N  P  N  L  B  U  D
O  O  O  S  Q  L  R  M  E  T  I  S  I  P  M
R  K  C  E  M  O  O  N  I  H  I  Q  F  W  W
H  U  R  T  C  N  I  B  P  A  S  G  Z  T  G
E  E  I  Y  O  B  O  O  I  V  E  W  E  T  X
S  L  T  C  M  D  S  E  C  N  R  T  U  N  R
U  E  Y  O  Y  A  I  M  E  K  U  E  L  Y  S
S  T  R  G  B  S  T  H  R  O  M  B  U  S  Q
E  H  Z  A  M  S  A  L  P  N  D  Z  P  O  N
T  E  N  H  F  P  D  A  P  M  E  E  I  B  W
E  W  B  P  H  K  B  O  N  C  K  W  X  V  J
```

AIDS	Factor	Phagocytes
Anemia	Fibrin	Plasma
Antibody	Hematocrit	Recipient
Antigen	Hemoglobin	Rhesus
Basophil	Heparin	Serum
Donor	Leukemia	Thrombin
Embolus	Leukocytes	Thrombus
Erythrocytes	Monocyte	Type

❓ DID YOU KNOW?

- In the second it takes to turn the page of a book, you will lose about 3 million red blood cells. During that same second, your bone marrow will have produced the same number of new ones.
- There is enough iron in a human to make a small nail.
- Each whole blood donation can help as many as three people. One unit is divided into three parts: red blood cells, platelets, and plasma.
- Statistics show that 25% or more of us will require blood at least once in our lifetime.

BLOOD

Fill in the crossword puzzle.

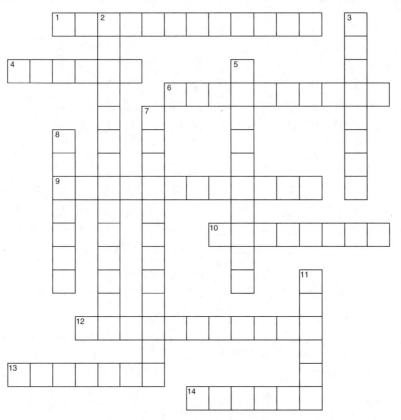

ACROSS
1. Abnormally high WBC count
4. Final stage of clotting process
6. Oxygen-carrying mechanism of blood
9. To engulf and digest microbes
10. Stationary blood clot
12. RBC
13. Circulating blood clot
14. Liquid portion of blood

DOWN
2. Type O (two words)
3. Substances that stimulate the body to make antibodies
5. Type of leukocyte
7. Platelets
8. Prevents clotting of blood
11. Inability of the blood to carry sufficient oxygen

CHECK YOUR KNOWLEDGE

Multiple Choice

Select the best answer.

1. The two primary functions of blood are:
   a. Communication and integration of body functions
   b. Transportation and protection
   c. Elimination of wastes and regulation of body temperature
   d. Synthesis of chemicals and regulation of acid-base balance

2. Which of the following is *not* a formed element?
   a. Neutrophils
   b. Blood serum
   c. Platelets
   d. Erythrocytes

3. Which of the following is an agranulocyte?
   a. Monocyte
   b. Neutrophil
   c. Eosinophil
   d. Basophil

4. Without adequate _____ in the diet, the body cannot manufacture enough hemoglobin.
   a. Iron
   b. Calcium
   c. Sodium
   d. Vitamin C

5. All of the following are necessary for successful blood clotting *except:*
   a. Platelets
   b. Prothrombin
   c. Fibrin
   d. Heparin

6. The function of white blood cells is to:
   a. Defend the body from microorganisms invading the body
   b. Transport oxygen to the cells
   c. Play an essential part in blood clotting
   d. None of the above

7. A blood clot that is stationary and stays in the place where it formed is called a(n):
   a. Thrombus
   b. Embolus
   c. Anticoagulant
   d. Coumadin

8. An *antibody* may be defined as:
   a. A substance made by the body in response to stimulation by an antigen
   b. A substance that reacts with the antigen that stimulated its formation
   c. A substance that causes antigens to agglutinate
   d. All of the above

9. Which blood type is considered the *universal recipient?*
   a. A-negative
   b. B-positive
   c. AB-positive
   d. O-negative

10. Erythroblastosis fetalis is now avoidable by treating all Rh-negative mothers who carry an Rh-positive baby with a protein marketed as:
    a. Rhesus immune treatment
    b. RhoGAM
    c. PolyHeme
    d. None of the above

Matching

Select the most correct answer from column B for each statement in column A. (Only one answer is correct.)

Column A

11. _____ Plasma

12. _____ Erythrocytes

13. _____ Myeloid tissue

14. _____ Hematocrit

15. _____ Buffy coat

16. _____ Eosinophils

17. _____ Leukocytosis

18. _____ Polycythemia

19. _____ Leukopenia

20. _____ Agglutinate

Column B

a. RBC volume
b. Abnormally high WBC count
c. Allergy protection
d. Liquid portion of blood
e. Abnormally high RBC count
f. No nuclei
g. WBCs and platelets
h. Hematopoiesis
i. Abnormally low WBC count
j. Clump

HUMAN BLOOD CELLS

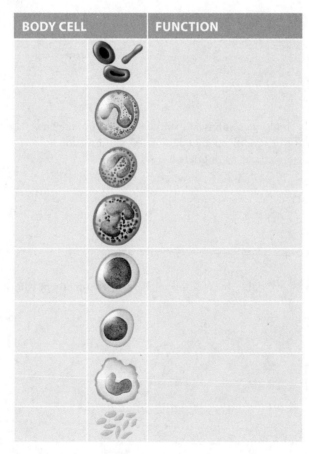

BODY CELL	FUNCTION

BLOOD TYPING

Using the key below, draw the appropriate reaction with the donor's blood in the circles.

Recipient's blood		Reactions with donor's blood			
RBC antigens	Plasma antibodies	Donor type O	Donor type A	Donor type B	Donor type AB
None (Type O)	Anti-A Anti-B	◯	◯	◯	◯
A (Type A)	Anti-B	◯	◯	◯	◯
B (Type B)	Anti-A	◯	◯	◯	◯
AB (Type AB)	(none)	◯	◯	◯	◯

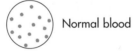 Normal blood   Agglutinated blood

CHAPTER 13

Cardiovascular System

The heart is actually two pumps: one to move blood to the lungs, the other to push it out into the body. These two functions seem rather elementary in comparison to the complex and numerous functions performed by most of the other body organs, and yet, if either of these pumps stop, within a few short minutes all life ceases.

The heart is divided into two upper compartments, called *atria,* that serve as receiving chambers, and two lower compartments, called *ventricles,* that serve as discharging chambers. By the time a person reaches age 45, approximately 300,000 tons of blood will have passed through these chambers to be circulated to the blood vessels. These vessels— arteries, veins, and capillaries—serve different functions. Arteries carry blood from the heart, veins carry blood to the heart, and capillaries are exchange vessels or connecting links between the arteries and veins. This closed system of circulation provides distribution of blood to the whole body (systemic circulation) and to specific regions, such as pulmonary circulation or hepatic portal circulation.

Blood pressure is the force of blood in the vessels. This force is highest in arteries and lowest in veins. Normal blood pressure varies among individuals and depends on the volume of blood in the arteries. The larger the volume of blood in the arteries, the more pressure is exerted on the walls of the arteries, and the higher the arterial pressure. Conversely, the less blood in the arteries, the lower the blood pressure.

A functional cardiovascular system is vital for survival, because without circulation, tissues would lack a supply of oxygen and nutrients. Waste products would begin to accumulate and could become toxic. Your review of this system will provide you with an understanding of the complex transportation mechanism of the body that is necessary for survival.

TOPICS FOR REVIEW

Before progressing to Chapter 14, you should have an understanding of the structure and function of the heart and blood vessels. Your review should include a study of systemic, pulmonary, hepatic portal, and fetal circulations and should conclude with a thorough understanding of blood pressure and pulse.

HEART

Fill in the blanks.

1. Rhythmic compression of the heart combined with effective artificial respiration is known as
   _____.

2. The _____ _____ divides the heart into right and left sides between the atria.

3. The _____ are the two upper chambers of the heart.

4. The _____ are the two lower chambers of the heart.

5. The cardiac muscle tissue is referred to as the _____.

6. Inflammation of the heart lining is _____.

7. The two AV valves are _____ and _____.

8. _____ _____ involves the movement of blood from the right ventricle to the lungs.

9. An occlusion of a coronary artery is known as a(n) _____.

10. _____ _____ occurs when heart muscle cells are deprived of oxygen and become damaged or die.

11. The pacemaker of the heart is the _____ node.

12. A normal ECG tracing has three characteristic waves. They are _____, _____, and _____ waves.

13. _____ begins just before the relaxation phase of cardiac muscle activity noted on an ECG.

Choose the correct term and write the letter in the space next to the appropriate definition below.

a. Pericardium
b. Severe chest pain
c. Thrombus
d. Pulmonary
e. Heart block
f. Ventricles
g. Systemic
h. Coronary arteries
i. Systole
j. Depolarization
k. Atria
l. Apex
m. Epicardium

14. _____ Covering of heart

15. _____ Receiving chambers

16. _____ Circulation from left ventricle throughout body

17. _____ Blood clot

18. _____ Semilunar valve

19. _____ Discharging chambers

20. _____ Supplies oxygen to heart muscle

21. _____ Angina pectoris

22. _____ Slow heart rate caused by blocked impulses

23. _____ Contraction of the heart

24. _____ Electrical activity associated with ECG

25. _____ Blunt-pointed lower edge of heart

26. _____ Visceral pericardium

➡ *If you had difficulty with this section, review pages 283-292.*

CARDIAC OUTPUT

Circle the best answer.

27. Cardiac output is the volume of blood pumped by one atrium (*per minute* or *per second*).

28. The (*sympathetic* or *parasympathetic*) system of the ANS decreases the heart rate.

29. The (*higher* or *lower*) the venous return, the higher the stroke volume.

30. The strength of myocardial (*contraction* or *relaxation*) helps determine stroke volume.

31. The average cardiac output in a normal, resting adult is (*5* or *7*) liters.

➡ *If you had difficulty with this section, review pages 292-294.*

BLOOD VESSELS—ROUTES OF CIRCULATION

Matching

Match the term on the left with the proper selection on the right.

32. _____ Arteries

33. _____ Veins

34. _____ Capillaries

35. _____ Tunica externa

36. _____ Precapillary sphincters

37. _____ Superior vena cava

38. _____ Aorta

a. Smooth muscle cells that guard entrance to capillaries
b. Carry blood to the heart
c. Carry blood into venules
d. Carry blood away from the heart
e. Largest vein
f. Largest artery
g. Outermost layer of arteries and veins

Multiple Choice

Select the best answer.

39. The aorta carries blood out of the:
    a. Right atrium
    b. Left atrium
    c. Right ventricle
    d. Left ventricle
    e. None of the above

40. The superior vena cava returns blood to the:
    a. Left atrium
    b. Left ventricle
    c. Right atrium
    d. Right ventricle
    e. None of the above

41. Which one of the following vessel's walls are made up entirely of endothelial cells?
    a. Vein
    b. Capillary
    c. Artery
    d. Venule
    e. Arteriole

42. The _____ is made up of smooth muscle.
    a. Tunica media
    b. Tunica adventitia
    c. Tunica intima
    d. Endothelium
    e. Myocardium

43. The _____ function as exchange vessels.
    a. Venules
    b. Capillaries
    c. Arteries
    d. Arterioles
    e. Veins

44. Blood returns from the lungs during pulmonary circulation via the:
    a. Pulmonary artery
    b. Pulmonary veins
    c. Aorta
    d. Inferior vena cava

45. The hepatic portal circulation serves the body by:
    a. Removing excess glucose and storing it in the liver as glycogen
    b. Detoxifying blood
    c. Removing various poisonous substances present in the blood
    d. All of the above

46. The structure used to bypass the liver in fetal circulation is the:
    a. Foramen ovale
    b. Ductus venosus
    c. Ductus arteriosus
    d. Umbilical vein

47. The foramen ovale serves the fetal circulation by:
    a. Connecting the aorta and the pulmonary artery
    b. Shunting blood from the right atrium directly into the left atrium
    c. Bypassing the liver
    d. Bypassing the lungs

48. The structure used to connect the aorta and pulmonary artery in fetal circulation is the:
    a. Ductus arteriosus
    b. Ductus venosus
    c. Aorta
    d. Foramen ovale

49. Which of the following is *not* an artery?
    a. Femoral
    b. Popliteal
    c. Coronary
    d. Inferior vena cava

50. Which of the following has valves to assist the blood flow?
    a. Veins
    b. Arteries
    c. Capillaries
    d. Arterioles

➡ *If you had difficulty with this section, review pages 294-302.*

HEMODYNAMICS—PULSE

True or False

If the statement is true, write "T" in the answer blank. If the statement is false, correct the statement by circling the incorrect term and writing the correct term in the answer blank.

51. _____ Blood pressure is highest in the veins and lowest in the arteries.

52. _____ The difference between two blood pressures is referred to as blood pressure deficit.

53. _____ If the blood pressure in the arteries were to decrease so that it became equal to the average pressure in the arterioles, circulation would increase.

54. _____ A stroke is often the result of low blood pressure.

55. _____ Massive hemorrhage increases blood pressure.

56. _____ Blood pressure is the volume of blood in the vessels.

57. _____ Both the strength and the rate of heartbeat affect cardiac output and blood pressure.

58. _____ The diameter of the arterioles helps to determine how much blood drains out of arteries into arterioles.

59. _____ A stronger heartbeat tends to decrease blood pressure, and a weaker heartbeat tends to increase it.

60. _____ The systolic pressure is the pressure while the ventricles relax.

61. _____ The diastolic pressure is the pressure while the ventricles contract.

62. _____ The pulse is a vein expanding and then recoiling.

63. _____ The radial artery is located at the wrist.

64. _____ The common carotid artery is located in the neck along the front edge of the sternocleidomastoid muscle.

65. _____ The artery located at the bend of the elbow and used for locating the pulse is the dorsalis pedis.

➔ *If you had difficulty with this section, review pages 302-307.*

UNSCRAMBLE THE WORDS

Unscramble the circled letters and fill in the statement.

66. **S T M E S Y C I**

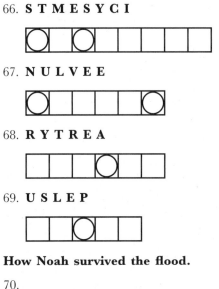

67. **N U L V E E**

68. **R Y T R E A**

69. **U S L E P**

How Noah survived the flood.

70.

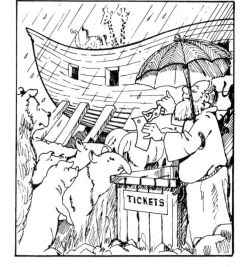

APPLYING WHAT YOU KNOW

71. Mr. Rainey was experiencing angina pectoris. His doctor suggested a surgical procedure that would require the removal of a vein from another region of his body. This vein would then be used to bypass a partial blockage in his coronary arteries. What is this procedure called?

72. Phil has heart block. His electrical impulses are being blocked from reaching the ventricles. An electrical device that causes ventricular contractions at a rate necessary to maintain circulation is being considered as possible treatment for his condition. What is this device called?

73. Mrs. Haygood was diagnosed with an acute case of endocarditis. What is the real danger of this diagnosis?

74. Dan returned from surgery in stable condition. The nurse noted that each time she took Dan's pulse and blood pressure, the pulse became higher and the blood pressure lower than the last time. What might be the cause?

75. WORD FIND

Can you find 15 terms from this chapter in the box of letters? Words may be spelled top to bottom, bottom to top, right to left, left to right, or diagonally.

```
Y  H  Y  S  I  S  O  B  M  O  R  H  T  A  R
L  A  C  I  L  I  B  M  U  O  A  Y  N  I  Y
E  E  S  Y  S  T  E  M  I  C  C  G  D  E  U
M  V  E  N  U  L  E  D  D  C  I  X  M  D  I
E  Y  M  U  I  R  T  A  R  N  L  E  C  G  Y
N  O  I  T  A  Z  I  R  A  L  O  P  E  D  N
U  D  L  A  T  R  O  P  C  I  T  A  P  E  H
S  I  U  K  M  U  E  T  O  E  S  L  U  P  U
R  P  N  F  Y  C  B  E  D  R  A  L  Z  P  J
D  S  A  H  T  I  T  V  N  L  I  I  B  D  W
Q  U  R  O  I  V  A  Q  E  O  D  A  K  R  K
K  C  R  M  P  G  A  I  G  N  D  D  Z  Y  J
Y  I  Y  R  I  N  E  A  F  Z  L  Q  S  P  X
S  R  M  I  C  C  Q  O  A  W  U  N  H  O  K
P  T  A  V  H  H  Z  L  H  I  J  J  X  K  Z
```

Angina pectoris	ECG	Systemic
Apex	Endocardium	Thrombosis
Atrium	Hepatic portal	Tricuspid
Depolarization	Pulse	Umbilical
Diastolic	Semilunar	Venule

❓ DID YOU KNOW?

- Your heart pumps more than 5 quarts of blood every minute, or 2,000 gallons a day.
- Every pound of excess fat contains some 200 miles of additional capillaries to push blood through each minute.
- If laid out in a straight line, the average adult's circulatory system would be nearly 60,000 miles long—enough to circle the earth 2.5 times!
- People who have an optimistic attitude as opposed to a pessimistic attitude suffer fewer strokes and heart attacks and have a 55% less chance of suffering cardiovascular diseases.

CARDIOVASCULAR SYSTEM

Fill in the crossword puzzle.

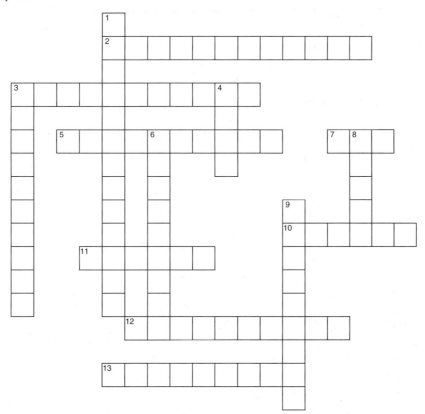

ACROSS

2. Inflammation of the lining of the heart
3. Bicuspid valve (2 words)
5. Inner layer of pericardium
7. Cardiopulmonary resuscitation (abbreviation)
10. Carries blood away from the heart
11. Upper chamber of the heart
12. Lower chambers of the heart
13. SA node

DOWN

1. Unique blood circulation through the liver (2 words)
3. Muscular layer of the heart
4. Carries blood to the heart
6. Tiny artery
8. Heart rate
9. Carries blood from arterioles to venules

CHECK YOUR KNOWLEDGE

Multiple Choice

Select the best answer.

1. Heart sounds are most easily heard by placing a stethoscope:
   a. Directly over the apex of the heart
   b. Over the space between the first and second ribs
   c. Over the upper portion of the mediastinum
   d. None of the above

2. The valve located between the right atrium and ventricle is the:
   a. Bicuspid
   b. Aortic semilunar valve
   c. Tricuspid
   d. Pulmonary semilunar valve

3. Blood rich in oxygen returns from the lungs and enters the left atrium of the heart through the:
   a. Aorta
   b. Pulmonary veins
   c. Superior vena cava
   d. Pulmonary artery

4. Heart block is often successfully treated by:
   a. Implanting an artificial pacemaker
   b. Coronary bypass surgery
   c. Angioplasty
   d. None of the above

5. The outermost layer of the arteries and veins is the:
   a. Tunica externa
   b. Tunica media
   c. Tunica intima
   d. Endothelium

6. An electrocardiogram (ECG):
   a. Is a graphic record of the heart's electrical activity
   b. Records damage to cardiac muscle tissue that affects the heart's conduction system
   c. Has three deflections known as the *P wave*, the *QRS complex*, and the *T wave*
   d. All of the above

7. The blood pressure gradient is:
   a. The pressure against the arteries during contraction
   b. The pressure against the arteries at rest
   c. Vitally involved in keeping the blood flowing
   d. The artery expanding and then recoiling alternately

8. The structure(s) unique to fetal circulation is the:
   a. Ductus venosus
   b. Ductus arteriosus
   c. Foramen ovale
   d. All of the above

9. *Stroke volume* refers to the:
   a. Volume of blood pumped by one ventricle per minute
   b. Flow of blood into the cardiac veins
   c. Volume of blood ejected from the ventricles during each beat
   d. Flow of blood into the coronary sinus

10. A structural feature *not* present in arteries and unique to veins is:
    a. Tunica intima
    b. Tunica media
    c. One-way valves
    d. Tunica adventitia

Matching

Select the most correct answer from column B for each statement in column A. (Only one answer is correct.)

Column A

11. _____ Atria

12. _____ Endocardium

13. _____ Pericardium

14. _____ Superior vena cava

15. _____ Aorta

16. _____ Bundle of His

17. _____ Ventricles

18. _____ Central venous pressure

19. _____ Pulse

20. _____ Diastole

Column B

a. Right atrium
b. AV bundle
c. Discharging chambers
d. Radial artery
e. Ventricles relaxed
f. Receiving chambers
g. Lining of heart
h. Covering of heart
i. Vein
j. Artery

THE HEART

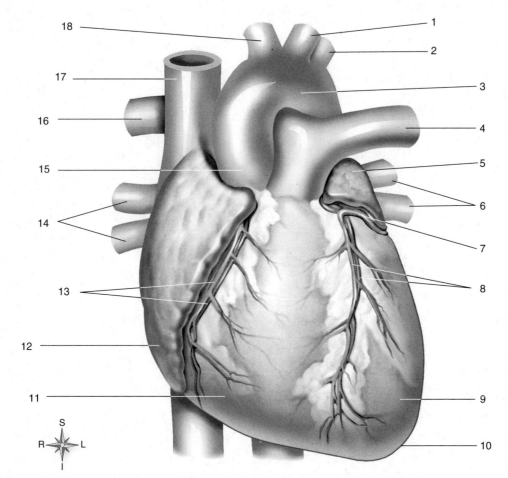

1. _____

2. _____

3. _____

4. _____

5. _____

6. _____

7. _____

8. _____

9. _____

10. _____

11. _____

12. _____

13. _____

14. _____

15. _____

16. _____

17. _____

18. _____

CONDUCTION SYSTEM OF THE HEART

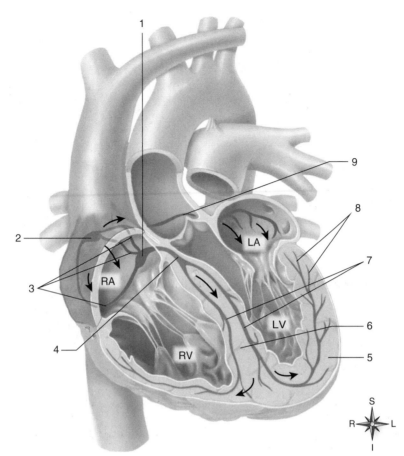

1. _____
2. _____
3. _____
4. _____
5. _____

6. _____
7. _____
8. _____
9. _____

FETAL CIRCULATION

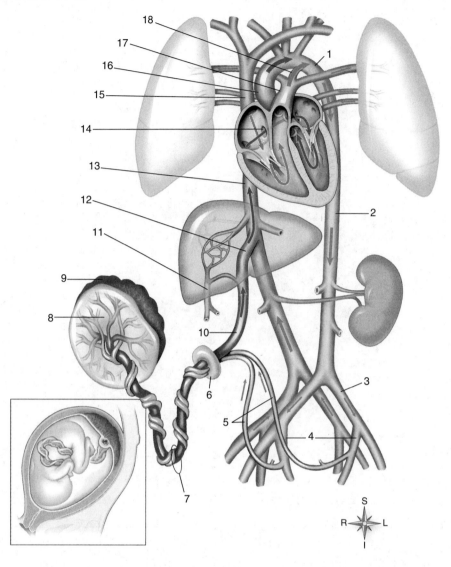

1. _____   10. _____

2. _____   11. _____

3. _____   12. _____

4. _____   13. _____

5. _____   14. _____

6. _____   15. _____

7. _____   16. _____

8. _____   17. _____

9. _____   18. _____

HEPATIC PORTAL CIRCULATION

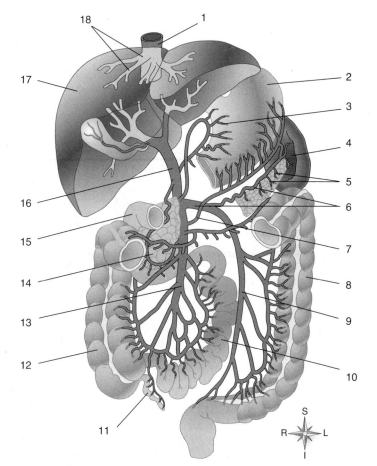

1. _____
2. _____
3. _____
4. _____
5. _____
6. _____
7. _____
8. _____
9. _____

10. _____
11. _____
12. _____
13. _____
14. _____
15. _____
16. _____
17. _____
18. _____

PRINCIPAL ARTERIES OF THE BODY

1. _____
2. _____
3. _____
4. _____
5. _____
6. _____
7. _____
8. _____
9. _____
10. _____
11. _____
12. _____
13. _____
14. _____
15. _____
16. _____
17. _____
18. _____
19. _____
20. _____
21. _____
22. _____
23. _____
24. _____
25. _____
26. _____
27. _____
28. _____
29. _____
30. _____

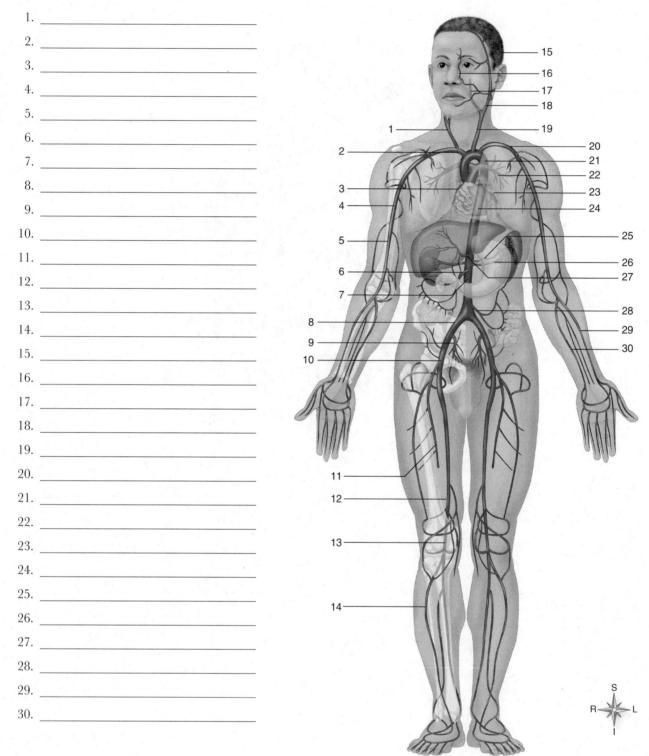

PRINCIPAL VEINS OF THE BODY

1. _____
2. _____
3. _____
4. _____
5. _____
6. _____
7. _____
8. _____
9. _____
10. _____
11. _____
12. _____
13. _____
14. _____
15. _____
16. _____
17. _____
18. _____
19. _____
20. _____
21. _____
22. _____
23. _____
24. _____
25. _____
26. _____
27. _____
28. _____
29. _____
30. _____
31. _____
32. _____
33. _____
34. _____
35. _____

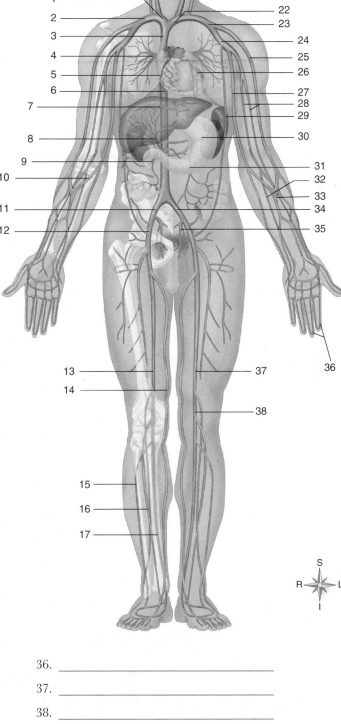

36. _____
37. _____
38. _____

NORMAL ECG DEFLECTIONS

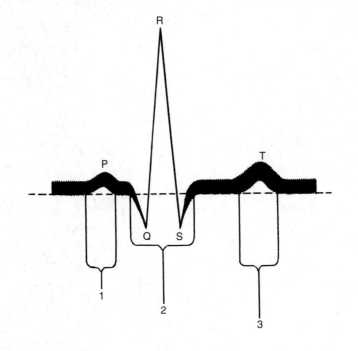

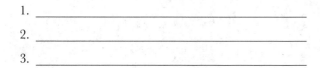

1. _____

2. _____

3. _____

14

Lymphatic System and Immunity

The lymphatic system is similar to the circulatory system. Lymph, like blood, flows through an elaborate route of vessels. In addition to lymphatic vessels, the lymphatic system consists of lymph nodes, lymph, and the spleen. Unlike the circulatory system, the lymphatic vessels do not form a closed circuit. Lymph flows only once through the vessels before draining into the general blood circulation. This system is a filtering mechanism for microorganisms and serves as a protective device against foreign invaders, such as cancer.

The immune system is the armed forces division of the body. Ready to attack at a moment's notice, the immune system defends us against the major enemies of the body: microorganisms, foreign transplanted tissue cells, and our own cells that have turned malignant.

The most numerous cells of the immune system are the lymphocytes. These cells circulate in the body's fluids seeking invading organisms and destroying them with powerful lymphotoxins, lymphokines, or antibodies.

Phagocytes, another large group of immune system cells, assist with the destruction of foreign invaders by a process known as *phagocytosis*. Neutrophils, monocytes, and connective tissue cells called *macrophages* use this process to surround unwanted microorganisms, ingest and digest them, and render them harmless to the body.

Another weapon that the immune system possesses is *complement*. Normally a group of inactive enzymes present in the blood, complement can be activated to kill invading cells by drilling holes in their cytoplasmic membranes, allowing fluid to enter the cell until it bursts.

Your review of this chapter will give you an understanding of how the body defends itself from the daily invasion of destructive substances.

TOPICS FOR REVIEW

Before progressing to Chapter 15, you should familiarize yourself with the functions of the lymphatic system, the immune system, and the major structures that make up these systems. Your review should include knowledge of lymphatic vessels, lymph nodes, lymph, antibodies, complement, and the development of B and T cells. Your study should conclude with an understanding of the differences in humoral and cell-mediated immunity.

THE LYMPHATIC SYSTEM

Fill in the blanks.

1. _____ is a fluid formed in the tissue spaces that will be transported by way of vessels to eventually reenter the circulatory system.

2. Blood plasma that has filtered out of capillaries into microscopic spaces between cells is called
   _____ _____.

3. The network of tiny blind-ended tubes distributed in the tissue spaces is called _____ _____.

4. Lymph eventually empties into two terminal vessels called the _____ _____
   _____ and the _____ _____.

5. The thoracic duct has an enlarged pouchlike structure called the _____ _____.

6. Lymph is filtered by moving through _____ _____, located in clusters along the pathway of lymphatic vessels.

7. Lymph enters the node through one or more _____ lymph vessels.

8. Lymph exits from the node through a single _____ lymph vessel.

➜ *If you had difficulty with this section, review pages 317-321.*

THYMUS—TONSILS—SPLEEN

Select the correct term from the options given and write the letter in the answer blank.

a. Thymus
b. Tonsils
c. Spleen

9. _____ Palatine, pharyngeal, and lingual are examples

10. _____ Largest lymphoid organ in the body

11. _____ Destroys worn-out red blood cells

12. _____ Located in the mediastinum

13. _____ Serves as a reservoir for blood

14. _____ T lymphocytes

15. _____ Largest at puberty

➡ *If you had difficulty with this section, review pages 321-322.*

THE IMMUNE SYSTEM

Match the term on the left with the proper selection on the right.

16. _____ Nonspecific immunity

17. _____ Mother's milk

18. _____ Specific immunity

19. _____ Artificial passive immunity

20. _____ Immunization

a. Natural passive immunity
b. Injection of antibodies
c. General protection
d. Artificial active exposure
e. Adaptive immunity

➡ *If you had difficulty with this section, review pages 322-325.*

IMMUNE SYSTEM MOLECULES AND ALLERGIES

Choose the term that applies to each of the following descriptions. Write the letter for the term in the appropriate answer blank.

a. Antibodies
b. Antigen
c. Allergy
d. Anaphylactic shock
e. Cytokines
f. Complement cascade
g. Complement
h. Humoral immunity
i. Combining site
j. Interferon

21. _____ Hypersensitivity of the immune system to harmless antigens

22. _____ Life-threatening allergic reaction

23. _____ Chemicals released from cells to act as direct agents of innate, nonspecific immunity

24. _____ Protein compounds normally present in the body

25. _____ Also known as *antibody-mediated immunity*

26. _____ Combines with antibody to produce humoral immunity

27. _____ Antibody

28. _____ Process of changing molecule shape slightly to expose binding sites

29. _____ Small protein compound that plays a significant role in producing innate immunity against viral infections

30. _____ Inactive proteins in blood

Circle the one that does **not** *belong.*

31. Antibody   Allergy   Protein compound   Combining site

32. Antigen   Invading cells   Antibody   Fever

33. Memory   Innate   Native   Genetic

34. Allergy   Complement   Anaphylactic shock   Histamine

35. Macrophage   Lysis   Inactive enzymes   Plasma proteins

➔ *If you had difficulty with this section, review pages 325-327.*

IMMUNE SYSTEM CELLS

Multiple Choice

Select the best answer.

36. The most numerous cells of the immune system are the:
    a. Monocytes
    b. Eosinophils
    c. Neutrophils
    d. Lymphocytes
    e. Complement

37. Which of the terms listed below usually occurs during the second stage of B cell development?
    a. Plasma cells
    b. Stem cells
    c. Antibodies
    d. Activated B cells
    e. Inactive B cells

38. Which one of the terms listed below occurs last in the immune process?
    a. Plasma cells
    b. Stem cells
    c. Antibodies
    d. Activated B cells
    e. Inactive B cells

39. Moderate exercise has been found to:
    a. Decrease white blood cells
    b. Increase white blood cells
    c. Decrease platelets
    d. Decrease red blood cells

40. Which one of the following is part of the cell membrane of B cells?
    a. Complement
    b. Antigens
    c. Antibodies
    d. Epitopes
    e. None of the above

41. Immature B cells have:
    a. Four types of defense mechanisms on their cell membrane
    b. Several kinds of defense mechanisms on their cell membrane
    c. One specific kind of defense mechanism on their cell membrane
    d. No defense mechanisms on their cell membrane

42. Activation of a B cell depends on the B cell coming in contact with:
    a. Complement
    b. Antibodies
    c. Lymphotoxins
    d. Lymphokines
    e. Antigens

43. The kind of cell that produces large numbers of antibodies is the:
    a. B cell
    b. Stem cell
    c. T cell
    d. Memory cell
    e. Plasma cell

44. Just one of these short-lived cells that make antibodies can produce _____ of them per second.
    a. 20
    b. 200
    c. 2,000
    d. 20,000

45. Which of the following statements is *not* true of memory cells?
    a. They produce large numbers of antibodies.
    b. They are found in lymph nodes.
    c. They develop into plasma cells.
    d. They can react with antigens.
    e. All of the above are true of memory cells.

46. T cell development begins in the:
    a. Lymph nodes
    b. Liver
    c. Pancreas
    d. Spleen
    e. Thymus

47. Human immunodeficiency virus (HIV) has its most obvious effects in:
    a. B cells
    b. Stem cells
    c. Plasma cells
    d. T cells

48. Interferon:
    a. Is produced by body cells within hours after infection by a virus
    b. Decreases the severity of many virus-related diseases
    c. Shows promise as an anticancer agent
    d. Has been shown to be effective in treating breast cancer
    e. All of the above

49. B cells function indirectly to produce:
    a. Humoral immunity
    b. Cell-mediated immunity
    c. Lymphotoxins
    d. Lymphokines

50. T cells function to produce:
    a. Humoral immunity
    b. Cell-mediated immunity
    c. Antibodies
    d. Memory cells

Fill in the blanks.

51. All lymphocytes that circulate in the tissues arise from primitive cells in the bone marrow called

    _____ _____.

52. The first stage of B cell development—transformation of stem cells into immature B cells—occurs in the
    _____ and the _____ _____ before birth but only in the _____ _____ in adults.

53. _____ _____ secrete copious amounts of antibody into the blood—nearly
    2,000 antibody molecules for every second they live.

54. T cells are lymphocytes that have undergone their first stage of development in the _____

    _____.

55. _____ blocks HIV's ability to reproduce within infected cells.

56. _____ is a disease caused by a retrovirus that enters the bloodstream and integrates into
    the DNA of T cell lymphocytes.

57. Like many viruses such as the common cold, HIV changes rapidly so the development of a
    _____ may not occur for several years.

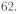 *If you had difficulty with this section, review pages 323 and 327-333.*

UNSCRAMBLE THE WORDS

Unscramble the circled letters and fill in the statement.

58. **N T C M P E O L E M**

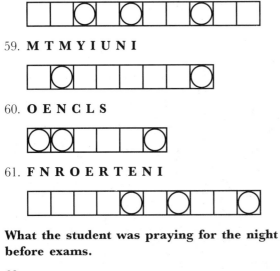

59. **M T M Y I U N I**

60. **O E N C L S**

61. **F N R O E R T E N I**

What the student was praying for the night before exams.

62.

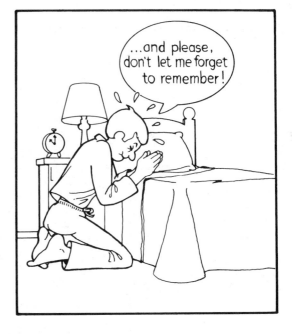

🖊 APPLYING WHAT YOU KNOW

63. Two-year-old baby Metcalfe was exposed to chickenpox. He had been a particularly sickly child, and so the doctor decided to give him a dose of interferon. What effect was the physician hoping for in baby Metcalfe's case?

64. Marcia was an intravenous drug user. She was recently diagnosed with Kaposi's sarcoma. What is another possible diagnosis?

65. Baby Phelps was born without a thymus gland. Immediate plans were made for a transplant to be performed. In the meantime, baby Phelps was placed in strict isolation. Why was this done?

66. WORD FIND

Can you find 14 terms from the chapter in the box of letters? Words may be spelled top to bottom, bottom to top, right to left, left to right, or diagonally.

```
I  N  F  L  A  M  M  A  T  O  R  Y  F  C  G
Q  N  L  O  Y  Z  O  C  C  P  A  O  F  S  X
M  W  T  A  A  M  N  J  X  Q  K  R  N  P  H
U  R  L  E  R  M  P  X  B  R  U  I  A  L  C
C  M  A  C  R  O  P  H  A  G  E  I  E  D  Z
X  M  N  D  K  F  M  N  O  T  U  C  R  N  M
A  E  O  R  E  Z  E  U  O  C  F  B  Y  E  B
Y  P  L  E  B  G  G  R  H  T  Y  T  S  E  D
Y  S  C  R  I  S  P  J  O  E  I  T  M  L  A
Z  M  O  T  J  X  E  T  O  N  A  E  E  P  X
T  O  N  S  I  L  S  S  U  M  Y  H  T  S  Y
W  A  O  C  J  N  I  M  W  K  O  Z  E  N  D
D  W  M  K  W  R  M  O  I  P  S  H  Y  B  G
F  H  W  U  J  I  Z  F  V  D  Z  L  Y  T  X
```

Acquired	Interferon	Proteins
Antigen	Lymph	Spleen
Humoral	Lymphocytes	Thymus
Immunity	Macrophage	Tonsils
Inflammatory	Monoclonal	

❓ DID YOU KNOW?

- There are more living organisms on the skin of a single human being than there are human beings on the surface of the earth.
- According to the Centers for Disease Control, 18 million courses of antibiotics are prescribed for the common cold in the United States per year. Research shows that colds are caused by viruses. Fifty million unnecessary antibiotics are prescribed for viral respiratory infections.
- The lymphatic system returns approximately 3.17 quarts (3 L) of fluid each day from the tissues to the circulatory system.

LYMPH AND IMMUNITY

Fill in the crossword puzzle.

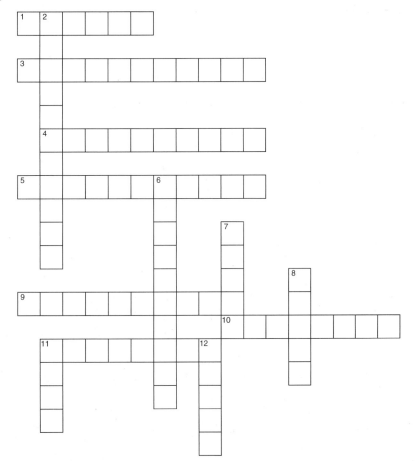

ACROSS

1. Largest lymphoid organ in the body
3. Connective tissue cells that are phagocytes
4. Protein compounds normally present in the body
5. Remain in reserve and then turn into plasma cells when needed (2 words)
9. Synthetically produced to fight certain diseases
10. Lymph exits the node through this lymph vessel
11. Lymph enters the node through these lymph vessels

DOWN

2. Secretes a copious amount of antibodies into the blood (2 words)
6. Inactive proteins
7. Family of identical cells descended from one cell
8. Type of lymphocyte (humoral immunity—2 words)
11. Immune deficiency disorder
12. Type of lymphocyte (cell-mediated immunity—2 words)

CHECK YOUR KNOWLEDGE

Multiple Choice

Select the best answer.

1. Which of the following is true about both lymphatic and blood capillaries?
   a. Both types of vessels are microscopic and are formed from sheets of endothelium.
   b. The movement and route of blood and lymph are identical.
   c. Both lymph and blood terminate in the same veins.
   d. All of the above are true.

2. The spleen:
   a. Is the largest lymphoid organ in the body
   b. Has a limited blood supply
   c. Is located in the upper right quadrant of the abdomen lateral to the stomach
   d. All of the above

3. Lymph nodes are responsible for:
   a. Defense
   b. White blood cell formation
   c. Biological filtration
   d. All of the above

4. Which of the following is *not* true regarding lymph vessels?
   a. Lymph enters the node through four afferent lymph vessels.
   b. Lymph exits the node through four efferent vessels.
   c. Once lymph enters the node, it "percolates" slowly through spaces called *sinuses*.
   d. Lymph from the breast drains into many different and widely placed nodes.

5. The thymus is:
   a. Largest at puberty
   b. A source of lymphocytes before birth
   c. Replaced by a process called *involution*
   d. All of the above

6. Which of the following is *not* an example of tonsils?
   a. Palatine
   b. Humoral
   c. Pharyngeal
   d. Lingual

7. Active immunity occurs when:
   a. Immunity to a disease that has developed in another individual is transferred to someone not previously immune
   b. An infant receives antibodies in her mother's milk
   c. Immunity is inherited
   d. A vaccination confers immunity

8. The function of T cells is to:
   a. Produce cell-mediated immunity
   b. Kill infected cells by releasing a substance that poisons cells
   c. Release chemicals that attract and activate macrophages to kill cells by phagocytosis
   d. All of the above

9. Which of the following is an example of nonspecific immunity?
   a. Skin
   b. Tears and mucus
   c. Inflammation
   d. All of the above

10. In general, antibodies produce _____ immunity.
    a. Complement
    b. Phagocytic
    c. Humoral
    d. Inherited

Matching

Select the most correct answer from column B for each statement in column A. (Only one answer is correct.)

Column A

11. _____ Lymph vessel

12. _____ Thymus

13. _____ Nonspecific immunity

14. _____ Specific immunity

15. _____ Protein compounds in the body

16. _____ Antigen hypersensitivity

17. _____ Antibody-mediated immunity

18. _____ Cytokines

19. _____ Synthetic treatment for viral infections

20. _____ Phagocytes

Column B

a. Humoral
b. Allergy
c. Interferon
d. T cells
e. Efferent
f. Macrophages
g. Antibodies
h. Adaptive immunity
i. Phagocytosis
j. Interleukins

PRINCIPAL ORGANS OF THE LYMPHATIC SYSTEM

1. _____
2. _____
3. _____
4. _____
5. _____
6. _____
7. _____
8. _____
9. _____
10. _____
11. _____
12. _____
13. _____

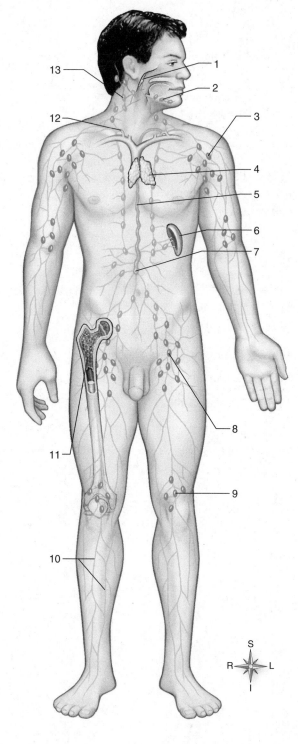

Respiratory System

As you sit reviewing this system, your body needs 16 quarts of air per minute. Walking requires 24 quarts of air per minute, and running requires 50 quarts per minute. The respiratory system provides the air necessary for you to perform your daily activities and eliminates the waste gases from the air that you breathe. Take a deep breath, and think of the air as entering some 250 million tiny air sacs similar in appearance to clusters of grapes. These microscopic air sacs expand to let air in and contract to force it out. These tiny sacs, alveoli, are the functioning units of the respiratory system. They provide the necessary volume of oxygen and eliminate carbon dioxide 24 hours a day.

Air enters either through the mouth or the nasal cavity. It next passes through the pharynx, past the epiglottis, and then through the glottis and the rest of the larynx. It then continues down the trachea, into the bronchi to the bronchioles, and finally through the alveoli. The reverse occurs for expelled air.

The exchange of gases between air in the lungs and in the blood is known as *external respiration*. The exchange of gases that occurs between the blood and the cells of the body is known as *internal respiration*. By constantly supplying adequate oxygen and by removing carbon dioxide as it forms, the respiratory system helps to maintain an environment conducive to maximum cell efficiency.

Your review of this system is necessary to provide you with an understanding of this essential homeostatic mechanism.

TOPICS FOR REVIEW

Before progressing to Chapter 16, you should have an understanding of the structure and function of the organs of the respiratory system. Your review should include knowledge of the mechanisms responsible for both internal and external respiration. Your study should conclude with knowledge of the volumes of air exchanged in pulmonary ventilation and an understanding of how respiration is regulated.

STRUCTURAL PLAN—RESPIRATORY TRACTS—RESPIRATORY MUCOSA

Match the term with the definition.

a. Diffusion
b. Olfactory receptors
c. Alveoli
d. URI
e. Respiration

f. Respiratory mucosa
g. Upper respiratory tract
h. Lower respiratory tract
i. Cilia
j. Air distributor

1. _____ Function of respiratory system

2. _____ Pharynx

3. _____ Passive transport process responsible for actual exchange of gases

4. _____ Assists with the movement of mucus toward the pharynx

5. _____ Nasal mucosa

6. _____ Lines the tubes of the respiratory tree

7. _____ Terminal air sacs

8. _____ Trachea

9. _____ Head cold

10. _____ Homeostatic mechanism

Fill in the blanks.

The organs of the respiratory system are designed to perform two basic functions. They serve as a(n) (11) _____ _____ and as a(n) (12) _____ _____. In addition to the above, the respiratory system (13) _____, (14) _____, and (15) _____ the air we breathe. Respiratory organs include the (16) _____, (17) _____, (18) _____, (19) _____, (20) _____, and (21) _____. The respiratory system ends in millions of tiny, thin-walled sacs called (22) _____. (23) _____ of gases takes place in these sacs. Finally, (24)_____ _____ lines most of the air distribution tubes of the respiratory system. This membrane is covered by pseudostratified columnar epithelium rich in mucus-producing (25)_____ cells.

NOSE—PHARYNX—LARYNX

Circle the one that does not *belong.*

26. Nares	Septum	Oropharynx	Conchae
27. Conchae	Frontal	Maxillary	Sphenoidal
28. Oropharynx	Throat	5 inches	Epiglottis
29. Pharyngeal	Adenoids	Uvula	Nasopharynx
30. Middle ear	Tubes	Nasopharynx	Larynx
31. Voice box	Thyroid cartilage	Tonsils	Vocal cords
32. Palatine	Eustachian tube	Tonsils	Oropharynx
33. Pharynx	Epiglottis	Adam's apple	Voice box

Choose the correct term from the options given and write the letter in the answer blank.

a. Nose
b. Pharynx
c. Larynx

34. _____ Warms and humidifies air

35. _____ Air and food pass through here

36. _____ Sinuses

37. _____ Conchae

38. _____ Septum

39. _____ Tonsils

40. _____ Middle ear infections

41. _____ Epiglottis

➲ *If you had difficulty with this section, review pages 341-346.*

TRACHEA—BRONCHIAL TREE—ALVEOLI—LUNGS

Fill in the blanks.

42. The windpipe is more properly referred to as the _____.

43. _____ keeps the framework of the trachea almost noncollapsible.

44. _____ is a major cause of death in the United States and includes choking on food and other substances caught in the trachea.

45. The first branch or division of the trachea leading to the lungs is the _____ _____.

46. Each alveolar duct ends in several _____ _____.

47. The narrow part of each lung, up under the collarbone, is its _____.

48. The _____ covers the outer surface of the lungs and lines the inner surface of the rib cage.

49. Inflammation of the lining of the thoracic cavity is _____.

50. The presence of air in the intrapleural space on one side of the chest is a(n) _____.

➡ *If you had difficulty with this section, review pages 346-351.*

RESPIRATION—PULMONARY VENTILATION

True or False

If the statement is true, write "T" in the answer blank. If the statement is false, correct the statement by circling the incorrect term and writing the correct term in the answer blank.

51. _____ Diffusion is the process that moves air into and out of the lungs.

52. _____ For inspiration to take place, the diaphragm and other respiratory muscles relax.

53. _____ Diffusion is a passive process that results in movement up a concentration gradient.

54. _____ The exchange of gases that occurs between blood in systemic capillaries and the body cells is external respiration.

55. _____ Many pulmonary volumes can be measured as a person breathes into a spirometer.

56. _____ Ordinarily we take about 2 pints of air into our lungs.

57. _____ The amount of air normally breathed in and out with each breath is called tidal volume.

58. _____ The largest amount of air that one can breathe out in one expiration is called residual volume.

59. _____ The inspiratory reserve volume is the amount of air that can be forcibly inhaled after a normal inspiration.

Multiple Choice

Select the best answer.

60. The term that means the same thing as breathing is:
   a. Gas exchange
   b. Respiration
   c. Inspiration
   d. Expiration
   e. Pulmonary ventilation

61. Carbaminohemoglobin is formed when _____ binds to hemoglobin.
   a. Oxygen
   b. Amino acids
   c. Carbon dioxide
   d. Nitrogen
   e. None of the above

62. Most of the oxygen transported by the blood is:
    a. Dissolved in white blood cells
    b. Bound to white blood cells
    c. Bound to hemoglobin
    d. Bound to carbaminohemoglobin
    e. None of the above

63. Which of the following would *not* assist inspiration?
    a. Elevation of the ribs
    b. Elevation of the diaphragm
    c. Contraction of the diaphragm
    d. Chest cavity becomes longer from top to bottom

64. A young adult male would have a vital capacity of about _____ mL.
    a. 500
    b. 1,200
    c. 3,300
    d. 4,800
    e. 6,200

65. The amount of air that can be forcibly exhaled after expiring the tidal volume is known as the:
    a. Total lung capacity
    b. Vital capacity
    c. Inspiratory reserve volume
    d. Expiratory reserve volume
    e. None of the above

66. Which one of the following is correct?
    a. VC = TV − IRV + ERV
    b. VC = TV + IRV − ERV
    c. VC = TV + IRV × ERV
    d. VC = TV + IRV + ERV
    e. None of the above

➜ *If you had difficulty with this section, review pages 351-354.*

REGULATION OF VENTILATION—BREATHING PATTERNS

Match the term on the left with the proper selection on the right.

67. _____ Respiratory control centers

68. _____ Chemoreceptors

69. _____ Pulmonary stretch receptors

70. _____ Dyspnea

71. _____ Respiratory arrest

72. _____ Eupnea

73. _____ Hypoventilation

a. Difficult breathing
b. Located in carotid bodies
c. Slow and shallow respirations
d. Normal respiratory rate
e. Located in the brain stem
f. Failure to resume breathing following a period of apnea
g. Located throughout pulmonary airways and in the alveoli

➜ *If you had difficulty with this section, review pages 354-360.*

UNSCRAMBLE THE WORDS

Unscramble the circled letters and fill in the statement.

74. **S P U E L I R Y**

⬜ ◯ ⬜ ⬜ ◯ ⬜ ⬜ ⬜

75. **C R N B O S I T H I**

⬜ ⬜ ◯ ◯ ⬜ ⬜ ◯ ⬜ ⬜ ⬜

76. **S E S X P T I A I**

⬜ ⬜ ⬜ ◯ ◯ ⬜ ⬜ ◯ ⬜

77. **D D N E A O I S**

◯ ⬜ ⬜ ◯ ⬜ ◯ ⬜ ⬜

What Mona Lisa was to DaVinci.

78.

⬜ ⬜ ⬜ ⬜ ⬜ ⬜ ⬜ ⬜ ⬜ ⬜ ⬜

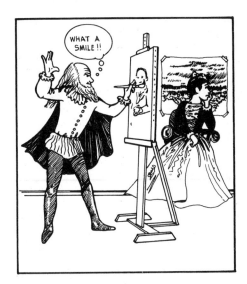

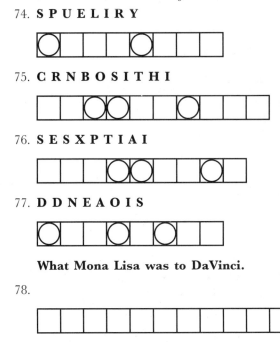

APPLYING WHAT YOU KNOW

79. Mr. Gorski is a heavy smoker. Recently he has noticed that when he gets up in the morning, he has a bothersome cough that brings up a large accumulation of mucus. This cough persists for several minutes and then leaves until the next morning. What is an explanation for this problem?

80. Michaela is 5 years old and is a mouth breather. She has had repeated episodes of tonsillitis and the pediatrician has suggested removal of her tonsils and adenoids. He has further suggested that the surgery would probably cure her mouth-breathing problem. Why is this a possibility?

81. WORD FIND

Can you find 14 terms from this chapter in the box of letters? Words may be spelled top to bottom, bottom to top, right to left, left to right, or diagonally.

```
N  K  S  A  Q  B  I  L  V  A  D  T  I  X  D
O  X  O  O  B  F  I  F  G  I  M  N  R  G  Y
I  G  N  X  W  D  E  E  F  L  B  A  U  T  S
T  B  K  Y  N  H  E  F  O  I  U  T  I  R  P
A  T  M  H  E  O  U  T  R  C  C  C  P  V  N
L  L  A  E  P  S  I  R  I  Z  A  A  N  F  E
I  P  T  M  I  H  G  T  I  P  R  F  P  C  A
T  U  B  O  G  Q  E  V  A  Q  O  R  V  N  W
N  L  N  G  L  R  J  C  C  R  T  U  P  D  C
E  M  U  L  O  V  L  A  U  D  I  S  E  R  E
V  O  V  O  T  A  N  G  J  E  D  P  Z  U  U
O  N  K  B  T  C  N  U  U  E  B  O  S  J  S
P  A  L  I  I  K  E  U  C  N  O  Z  K  N  A
Y  R  V  N  S  D  I  O  N  E  D  A  M  F  I
H  Y  O  M  L  O  A  Z  D  T  Y  M  N  L  K
```

Adenoids	Epiglottis	Residual volume
Carotid body	Hypoventilation	Surfactant
Cilia	Inspiration	URI
Diffusion	Oxyhemoglobin	Vital capacity
Dyspnea	Pulmonary	

❓ DID YOU KNOW?

- If the alveoli in our lungs were flattened out, they would cover a half of a tennis court.
- Sinusitis affects 37 million Americans, causing difficulty in breathing and chronic headaches.
- A person's nose and ears continue to grow throughout his or her life.
- Approximately a half a liter of water per day is lost through breathing.

RESPIRATORY SYSTEM

Fill in the crossword puzzle.

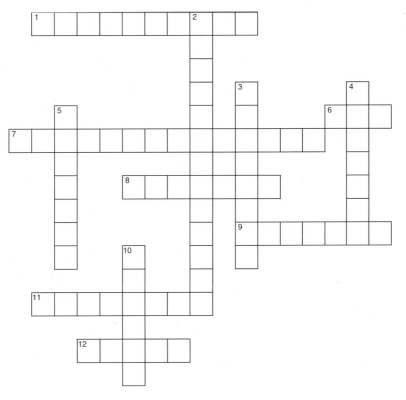

ACROSS

1. Device used to measure the amount of air exchanged in breathing
6. Expiratory reserve volume (abbreviation)
7. Sphenoidal (two words)
8. Terminal air sacs
9. Shelf-like structures that protrude into the nasal cavity
11. Inflammation of pleura
12. Respirations stop

DOWN

2. Surgical procedure to remove tonsils
3. Doctor who developed lifesaving technique
4. Windpipe
5. Trachea branches into right and left structures
10. Voice box

CHECK YOUR KNOWLEDGE

Multiple Choice

Select the best answer.

1. The exchange of gases between the air and blood is made possible by the process of:
   a. Diffusion
   b. Osmosis
   c. Filtration
   d. Pinocytosis

2. Which of the following is *not* a paranasal sinus?
   a. Frontal
   b. Temporal
   c. Maxillary
   d. Sphenoidal

3. The respiratory system serves the body as a(n):
   a. Air distributor
   b. Gas exchanger
   c. Important homeostatic mechanism
   d. All of the above

4. Select the correct pathway that air takes on the way to the lungs.
   a. Primary bronchi, secondary bronchi, alveolar sacs, alveolar ducts
   b. Primary bronchi, secondary bronchi, alveolar sacs, alveoli
   c. Primary bronchi, bronchioles, secondary bronchi, alveolar ducts
   d. Bronchioles, primary bronchi, secondary bronchi, alveoli

5. During expiration:
   a. The thoracic cavity decreases in size
   b. The lungs expand
   c. The diaphragm flattens out and contracts
   d. All of the above

6. The pleura:
   a. Covers the outer surface of the lungs and lines the inner surface of the rib cage
   b. Is an extensive, thin, moist, slippery membrane
   c. Is made up of two membranes known as the *parietal pleura* and *visceral pleura*
   d. All of the above

7. The exchange of gases that occurs between blood in tissue capillaries and the body cells is called:
   a. Internal respiration
   b. External respiration
   c. Vital capacity
   d. Inspiratory reserve volume

8. Residual volume is the:
   a. Amount of air that can be forcibly inspired over and above a normal inspiration
   b. Amount of air that can be forcibly exhaled after expiring the tidal volume
   c. Air that remains in the lungs after the most forceful expiration
   d. Largest amount of air that we can breathe out in one expiration

9. *Eupnea* is a term used to describe:
   a. Labored breathing
   b. A temporary stop in breathing
   c. Rapid respirations
   d. A normal respiratory rate

10. The respiratory control centers are located in the:
    a. Cerebrum
    b. Brain stem
    c. Cerebellum
    d. Thalamus

Matching

Select the most correct answer from column B for each statement in column A. (Only one answer is correct.)

Column A

11. _____ URI
12. _____ Lower respiratory tract
13. _____ External nares
14. _____ Voice box
15. _____ Trachea
16. _____ Spirometer
17. _____ Chemoreceptors
18. _____ Apnea
19. _____ Hypoventilation
20. _____ Apex

Column B

a. Nostrils
b. Used to measure air exchange
c. Carotid and aortic bodies
d. C-rings of cartilage
e. Head cold
f. Slow, shallow respirations
g. Larynx
h. Respiratory arrest
i. Chest cold
j. Lung

SAGITTAL VIEW OF THE HEAD AND NECK

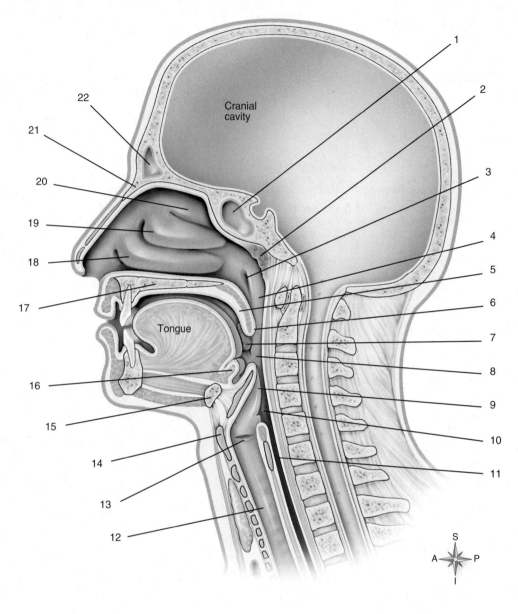

Cranial cavity

Tongue

S
A — P
I

1. _____   12. _____
2. _____   13. _____
3. _____   14. _____
4. _____   15. _____
5. _____   16. _____
6. _____   17. _____
7. _____   18. _____
8. _____   19. _____
9. _____   20. _____
10. _____   21. _____
11. _____   22. _____

RESPIRATORY ORGANS

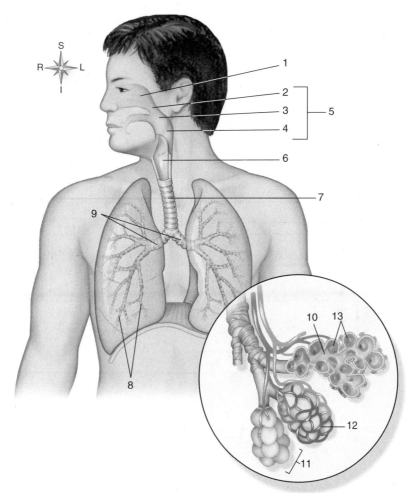

1. _____
2. _____
3. _____
4. _____
5. _____
6. _____
7. _____

8. _____
9. _____
10. _____
11. _____
12. _____
13. _____

PULMONARY VENTILATION VOLUMES

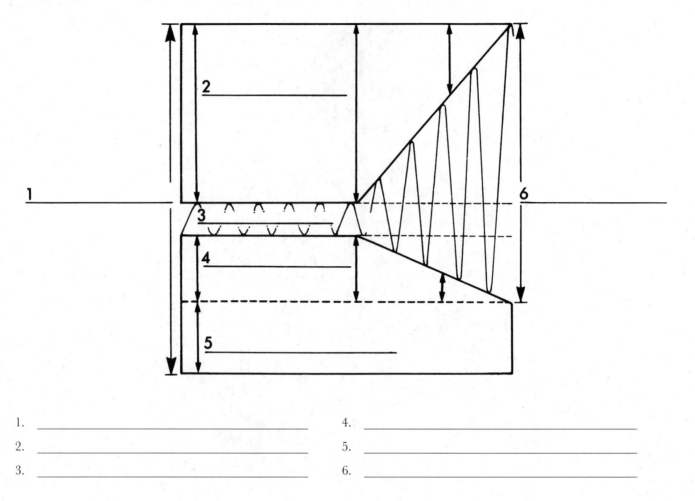

1. _____   4. _____

2. _____   5. _____

3. _____   6. _____

CHAPTER 16
Digestive System

Think of the last meal you ate. Imagine the different shapes, sizes, tastes, and textures that you so recently enjoyed. Think of those items circulating in your bloodstream in those same original shapes and sizes. Impossible? Of course. And because of this impossibility you will begin to understand and marvel at the close relationship of the digestive system to the circulatory system. It is the digestive system that changes our food, both mechanically and chemically, into a form that is acceptable to the blood and the body.

This change begins the moment you take the very first bite. Digestion starts in the mouth, where food is chewed and mixed with saliva. The food then moves down the pharynx and esophagus by peristalsis and enters the stomach. In the stomach it is churned and mixed with gastric juices to become chyme. The chyme goes from the stomach to the duodenum where it is further broken down chemically by intestinal fluids, bile, and pancreatic juice. Those secretions prepare the food for absorption all along the course of the small intestine.

Products that are not absorbed pass on through the entire length of the small intestine (duodenum, jejunum, ileum). From there they enter into the cecum of the large intestine, then the ascending colon, transverse colon, descending colon, sigmoid colon, into the rectum, and out the anus.

Products that are used in the cells undergo absorption. Absorption allows newly processed nutrients to pass through the walls of the digestive tract and into the bloodstream to be distributed to the cells.

Your review of this system will help you understand the mechanical and chemical processes necessary to convert food into energy sources and compounds necessary for survival.

TOPICS FOR REVIEW

Before progressing to Chapter 17, you should review the structure and function of all the organs of digestion. You should have an understanding of the process of digestion, both chemical and mechanical, and of the process of absorption.

OVERVIEW OF THE DIGESTIVE PROCESS—WALL OF THE DIGESTIVE SYSTEM

Fill in the blanks.

1. The organs of the digestive system form an irregularly shaped tube called the *alimentary canal,* or the
   _____ _____.

2. The churning of food in the stomach is an example of the _____ digestive process of food.

3. _____ breakdown occurs when digestive enzymes act on food as it passes through the digestive tract.

4. Waste material resulting from the digestive process is known as _____.

5. The process of ingested food being broken down into simpler nutrients is known as _____.

6. After the digestive processes have altered the physical and chemical composition of ingested food, the resulting nutrients are ready for the process of _____.

7. The digestive tract extends from the _____ to the _____.

8. The inside or hollow space within the alimentary canal is called the _____.

9. The inside layer of the digestive tract is the _____.

10. The connective tissue layer that lies beneath the lining of the digestive tract is the _____.

11. The muscularis contracts and moves food through the gastrointestinal tract by a process known as _____.

12. The outermost covering of the digestive tube is the _____.

13. The loops of the digestive tract are anchored to the posterior wall of the abdominal cavity by the _____.

Choose the correct term from the choices given and write the letter in the answer blank.

a. Main organ
b. Accessory organ

14. _____ Mouth

15. _____ Parotids

16. _____ Liver

17. _____ Stomach

18. _____ Cecum

19. _____ Esophagus

20. _____ Rectum

21. _____ Pharynx

22. _____ Appendix

23. _____ Teeth

24. _____ Gallbladder

25. _____ Pancreas

➲ *If you had difficulty with this section, review pages 366-370.*

MOUTH—TEETH—SALIVARY GLANDS

Select the best answer.

26. Which one of the following is *not* a part of the roof of the mouth?
    a. Uvula
    b. Palatine bones
    c. Maxillary bones
    d. Soft palate
    e. All of the above are part of the roof of the mouth

27. A thin membrane called the _____ attaches the tongue to the floor of the mouth.
    a. Filiform
    b. Fungiform
    c. Frenulum
    d. Root

28. The first baby tooth, on an average, appears at age:
    a. 2 months
    b. 1 year
    c. 3 months
    d. 1 month
    e. 6 months

29. The portion of the tooth that is covered with enamel is the:
    a. Pulp cavity
    b. Neck
    c. Root
    d. Crown
    e. None of the above

30. The wall of the pulp cavity is surrounded by:
    a. Enamel
    b. Dentin
    c. Cementum
    d. Connective tissue
    e. Blood and lymphatic vessels

31. A general term for mild, localized inflammation of the gums is:
    a. Periodontitis
    b. Dental caries
    c. Gingivitis
    d. Deciduitis

32. The leading cause of tooth loss among adults is:
    a. Dental caries
    b. Gingivitis
    c. Poor diet
    d. Periodontitis

33. The third molar appears between the ages of _____.
    a. 10 and 14
    b. 5 and 8
    c. 11 and 16
    d. 17 and 24
    e. None of the above

34. Which one of the following will *not* significantly reduce caries?
    a. Good dental health practices
    b. Regular flossing
    c. Regular and thorough brushing
    d. Eating a carrot or stick of celery instead of brushing

35. The ducts of the _____ glands open into the floor of the mouth.
    a. Sublingual
    b. Submandibular
    c. Parotid
    d. Carotid

36. The volume of saliva secreted per day is about:
    a. One-half pint
    b. One pint
    c. One liter
    d. One gallon

37. Mumps are an infection of the:
    a. Parotid gland
    b. Sublingual gland
    c. Submandibular gland
    d. Tonsils

38. Incisors are used during mastication to:
    a. Cut
    b. Pierce
    c. Tear
    d. Grind

39. Another name for the third molar is:
    a. Central incisor
    b. Wisdom tooth
    c. Canine
    d. Lateral incisor

40. After food has been chewed, it is formed into a small rounded mass called a:
    a. Moat
    b. Chyme
    c. Bolus
    d. Protease

➲ *If you had difficulty with this section, review pages 370-373.*

PHARYNX—ESOPHAGUS—STOMACH

Fill in the blanks.

The (41) _____ is a tubelike structure that functions as part of both respiratory and digestive systems. It connects the mouth with the (42) _____. The esophagus serves as a passageway for movement of food from the pharynx to the (43) _____. Food enters the stomach by passing through the muscular (44) _____ _____ at the end of the esophagus. Contraction of the stomach mixes the food thoroughly with the gastric juices and breaks it down into a semisolid mixture called (45) _____.

The three divisions of the stomach are the (46) _____, (47) _____, and (48) _____.

Food is held in the stomach by the (49) _____ _____ muscle long enough for partial digestion to occur. After food has been in the stomach for approximately 3 hours, the chyme will enter the (50) _____ _____.

Match the term with the correct definition.

a. Esophagus
b. Chyme
c. Peristalsis
d. Rugae
e. Triple therapy
f. Greater curvature
g. Hiatal hernia
h. Antacid
i. Acid indigestion
j. Lesser curvature

51. _____ Stomach folds

52. _____ Upper right border of stomach

53. _____ Condition that may result in backward movement or reflux of stomach contents into the lower portion of the esophagus

54. _____ 10-inch passageway

55. _____ Drug used to treat GERD

56. _____ Semisolid mixture of stomach contents

57. _____ Muscle contractions of the digestive system

58. _____ Used to heal ulcers and prevent recurrences

59. _____ Heartburn

60. _____ Lower left border of stomach

➜ *If you had difficulty with this section, review pages 373-376 and 378.*

SMALL INTESTINE—LIVER AND GALLBLADDER—PANCREAS

Select the best answer.

61. Which one is *not* part of the small intestine?
    a. Jejunum
    b. Ileum
    c. Cecum
    d. Duodenum

62. Which one of the following structures does *not* increase the surface area of the intestine for absorption?
    a. Plicae
    b. Rugae
    c. Microvilli
    d. Villi

63. The union of the cystic duct and hepatic duct forms the:
    a. Common bile duct
    b. Major duodenal papilla
    c. Minor duodenal papilla
    d. Pancreatic duct

64. Obstruction of the _____ will lead to jaundice.
    a. Hepatic duct
    b. Pancreatic duct
    c. Cystic duct
    d. None of the above

65. Each villus in the intestine contains a lymphatic vessel, or _____, that serves to absorb lipid or fat materials from the chyme.
    a. Plica
    b. Lacteal
    c. Villa
    d. Microvilli

66. The middle third of the duodenum contains the:
    a. Islets
    b. Fundus
    c. Body
    d. Rugae
    e. Major duodenal papilla

67. Most gastric and duodenal ulcers result from infection with the bacterium:
    a. Biaxin
    b. Metronidazole
    c. Prilosec
    d. *Helicobacter pylori*

68. The liver is an:
    a. Enzyme
    b. Endocrine organ
    c. Endocrine gland
    d. Exocrine gland

69. Fats in chyme stimulate the secretion of the hormone:
    a. Lipase
    b. Cholecystokinin
    c. Protease
    d. Amylase

70. The largest gland in the body is the:
    a. Pituitary
    b. Thyroid
    c. Liver
    d. Thymus

➔ *If you had difficulty with this section, review pages 376-380.*

LARGE INTESTINE—APPENDIX—PERITONEUM

True or False

If the statement is true, write "T" in the answer blank. If the statement is false, correct the statement by circling the incorrect term and writing the correct term in the answer blank.

71. _____ Bacteria in the large intestine are responsible for the synthesis of vitamin E needed for normal blood clotting.

72. _____ Villi in the large intestine absorb salts and water.

73. _____ If waste products pass rapidly through the large intestine, constipation results.

74. _____ The ileocecal valve opens into the sigmoid colon.

75. _____ The splenic flexure is the bend between the ascending colon and the transverse colon.

76. _____ The splenic colon is the S-shaped segment that terminates in the rectum.

77. _____ The appendix serves as a "breeding ground" for nonpathogenic intestinal bacteria.

78. _____ During movement through the large intestine, material that escapes digestion in the small intestine is acted on by intestinal microbiome, or "flora."

79. _____ The visceral layer of the peritoneum lines the abdominal cavity.

80. _____ The greater omentum is shaped like a fan and serves to anchor the small intestine to the posterior abdominal wall.

➔ *If you had difficulty with this section, review pages 380-383.*

DIGESTION—ABSORPTION

Select the best answer.

81. Which one of the following substances does *not* contain any enzymes?
    a. Saliva
    b. Bile
    c. Gastric juice
    d. Pancreatic juice
    e. Intestinal juice

82. Which one of the following is a simple sugar?
    a. Maltose
    b. Sucrose
    c. Lactose
    d. Glucose
    e. Starch

83. Cane sugar is the same as:
    a. Maltose
    b. Lactose
    c. Sucrose
    d. Glucose
    e. None of the above

84. Most of the digestion of carbohydrates takes place in the:
    a. Mouth
    b. Stomach
    c. Small intestine
    d. Large intestine

85. Fats are broken down into:
    a. Amino acids
    b. Simple sugars
    c. Fatty acids
    d. Disaccharides

➡ *If you had difficulty with this section, review pages 383-386.*

CHEMICAL DIGESTION

86. *Fill in the blank areas on the chart below.*

Digestive Juices and Enzymes	Substance Digested (or Hydrolyzed)	Resulting Product
Saliva		
1. Amylase	1.	1. Maltose (disaccharide)
Gastric Juice		
2. Protease (pepsin) plus hydrochloric acid	2. Proteins	2.
Pancreatic Juice		
3. Proteases (e.g., trypsin)	3. Proteins (intact or partially digested)	3.
4. Lipases	4.	4. Fatty acids, monoglycerides, and glycerol
5. Amylase	5.	5. Maltose
Intestinal Enzymes		
6. Peptidases	6.	6. Amino acids
7.	7. Sucrose	7. Glucose and fructose
8. Lactase	8.	8. Glucose and galactose (simple sugars)
9. Maltase	9. Maltose	9.

➡ *If you had difficulty with this section, review page 385.*

UNSCRAMBLE THE WORDS

Unscramble the circled letters and fill in the statement.

87. **S L B O U**

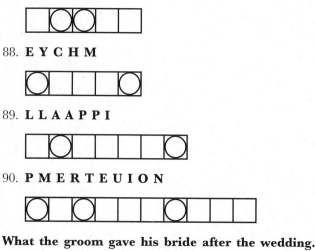

88. **E Y C H M**

89. **L L A A P P I**

90. **P M E R T E U I O N**

What the groom gave his bride after the wedding.

91.

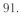 **APPLYING WHAT YOU KNOW**

92. Dan was a successful businessman, but he worked too hard and was always under great stress. His doctor cautioned him that if he did not alter his style of living he would be subject to hyperacidity. What could be the resulting condition of hyperacidity?

93. Baby Shearer has been regurgitating his bottle-feeding at every meal. The milk is curdled, but does not appear to be digested. He has become dehydrated, and so his mother is taking him to the pediatrician. Based on your textbook reading, what is a possible diagnosis?

94. Scott has gained a great deal of weight suddenly. He has also noticed that he is sluggish and always tired. What test might his physician order for him and for what reason?

95. WORD FIND

Can you find the 22 terms from the chapter in the box of letters? Words may be spelled top to bottom, bottom to top, right to left, left to right, or diagonally.

```
X M E T A B O L I S M X X W
R S D P E R I S T A L S I S
E V A M N O I T S E G I D R
E D E E U O Q T W Q O H N Q
Q Z H S R N I N T F E C E S
D H R E C C I T K C J A P E
Q W R N A T N V P Y R M P C
O C A T N R B A P R H O A I
U Y I E O W T A P A O T W D
B O D R L N P B F Q J S V N
N T S Y F I S L U M E E B U
W G J A L U V U N R N W O A
Q S N L X D U O D E N U M J
H C A V I T Y M U C O S A D
Y E A A P H V W S V C Q J C
```

Absorption	Emulsify	Mucosa
Appendix	Feces	Pancreas
Cavity	Fundus	Papillae
Crown	Heartburn	Peristalsis
Dentin	Jaundice	Stomach
Diarrhea	Mastication	Uvula
Digestion	Mesentery	
Duodenum	Metabolism	

❓ DID YOU KNOW?

- The liver performs more than 500 functions and produces more than 1,000 enzymes to handle the chemical conversions necessary for survival.
- The human stomach lining replaces itself every 3 days.
- Even if the stomach, the spleen, 75% of the liver, 80% of the intestines, one kidney, one lung, and virtually every organ from the pelvic and groin area are removed, the human body can still survive!
- Every day, approximately 11.5 L of digested food, liquids, and digestive juices flow through an individual's digestive system, but only 100 mL of that is lost in feces.

DIGESTIVE SYSTEM

Fill in the crossword puzzle.

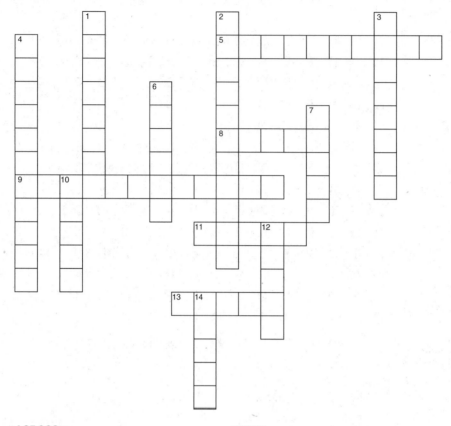

ACROSS

5. Digested food moves from intestine to blood
8. Semisolid mixture
9. Inflammation of the appendix
11. Rounded mass of food
13. Stomach folds

DOWN

1. Yellowish skin discoloration
2. Process of chewing
3. Fluid stools
4. Movement of food through digestive tract
6. Vomitus
7. Waste product of digestion
10. Intestinal folds
12. Open wound in digestive area acted on by acid juices
14. Prevents food from entering nasal cavities

CHECK YOUR KNOWLEDGE

Multiple Choice

Select the best answer.

1. The principal structure of the digestive system is an irregular tube, open at both ends, that is called the:
   a. Alimentary canal
   b. Oral cavity
   c. Colon
   d. Esophagus

2. Which of the following is *not* a layer of the digestive tract?
   a. Mucosa
   b. Muscularis
   c. Lumen
   d. Serosa

3. Which of the following is *not* a main organ of the digestive system?
   a. Liver
   b. Stomach
   c. Cecum
   d. Colon

4. Which of the following types of teeth have a cutting function during mastication?
   a. Canines
   b. Incisors
   c. Premolars
   d. Molars

5. Which of the following is an accurate description of the salivary glands?
   a. There are four pairs of salivary glands.
   b. Salivary amylase begins the chemical digestion of carbohydrates.
   c. They are located within the digestive tube.
   d. The submandibular glands are the ones involved when people have the mumps.

6. The act of swallowing moves a mass of food called a _____ from the mouth to the stomach.
   a. Dentin
   b. Bolus
   c. Chyme
   d. Frenulum

7. Stomach muscle contractions result in:
   a. Rugae
   b. Peristalsis
   c. Plicae
   d. None of the above

8. The stomach sphincter that keeps food from reentering the esophagus when the stomach contracts is known as the:
   a. Hiatal
   b. Pyloric
   c. Cardiac
   d. Fundus

9. Most of the chemical digestion occurs in the:
   a. Stomach
   b. Liver
   c. Duodenum
   d. Jejunum

10. The pancreas:
    a. Is both an endocrine and an exocrine gland
    b. Contains enzymes that digest proteins and fats only
    c. Contains an acid substance that elevates the pH of the gastric juice
    d. None of the above

Fill in the blanks.

11. Undigested and unabsorbed food materials enter the large intestine after passing through a sphincterlike structure called the _____ _____.

12. The subdivisions of the large intestine in the order in which food material or feces pass through them are cecum, ascending colon, transverse colon, descending colon, _____ _____, rectum, and anal canal.

13. The vermiform appendix is directly attached to the _____.

14. The _____ is an extension between the parietal and visceral layers of the peritoneum and is shaped like a giant, pleated fan.

15. Chewing, swallowing, peristalsis, and defecation are the main processes of _____ _____.

16. The end products of carbohydrate digestion are _____.

17. The end products of protein digestion are_____.

18. The end products of fat digestion are _____ and _____.

19. The process by which molecules of amino acids, glucose, fatty acids, and glycerol go from the inside of the intestines into the circulating fluids of the body is known as _____.

20. Three intestinal enzymes, _____, _____, and _____, digest disaccharides by changing them into monosaccharides.

DIGESTIVE ORGANS

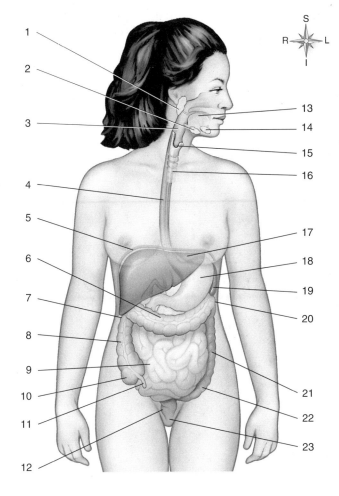

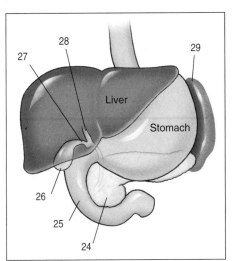

1. _____
2. _____
3. _____
4. _____
5. _____
6. _____
7. _____
8. _____
9. _____
10. _____
11. _____
12. _____
13. _____
14. _____
15. _____

16. _____
17. _____
18. _____
19. _____
20. _____
21. _____
22. _____
23. _____
24. _____
25. _____
26. _____
27. _____
28. _____
29. _____

TOOTH

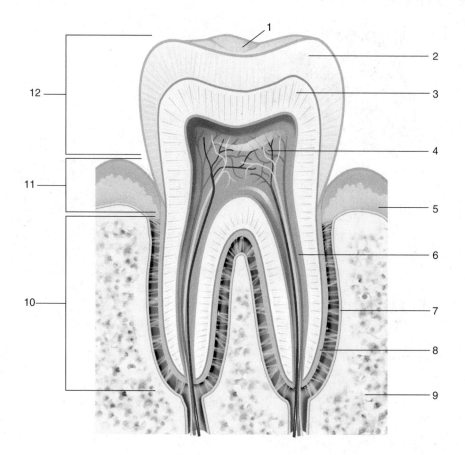

1. _____   7. _____

2. _____   8. _____

3. _____   9. _____

4. _____   10. _____

5. _____   11. _____

6. _____   12. _____

SALIVARY GLANDS

1. _____

2. _____

3. _____

4. _____

5. _____

STOMACH

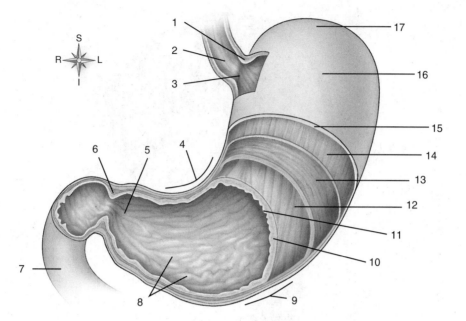

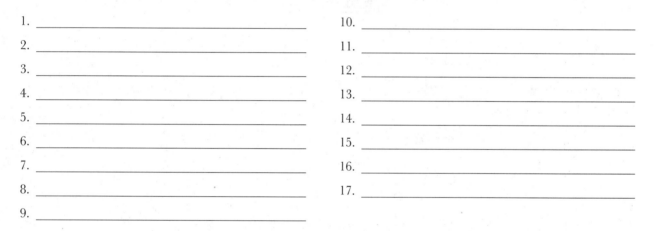

1. _____

2. _____

3. _____

4. _____

5. _____

6. _____

7. _____

8. _____

9. _____

10. _____

11. _____

12. _____

13. _____

14. _____

15. _____

16. _____

17. _____

GALLBLADDER AND BILE DUCTS

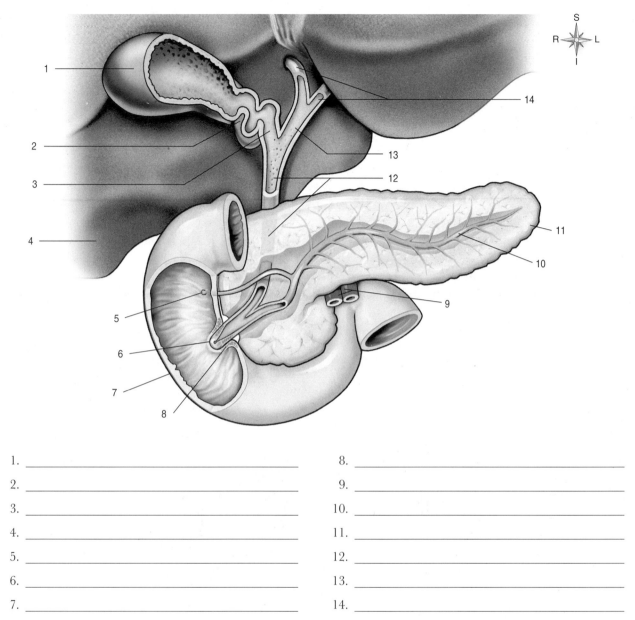

1. _____   8. _____

2. _____   9. _____

3. _____   10. _____

4. _____   11. _____

5. _____   12. _____

6. _____   13. _____

7. _____   14. _____

SMALL INTESTINE

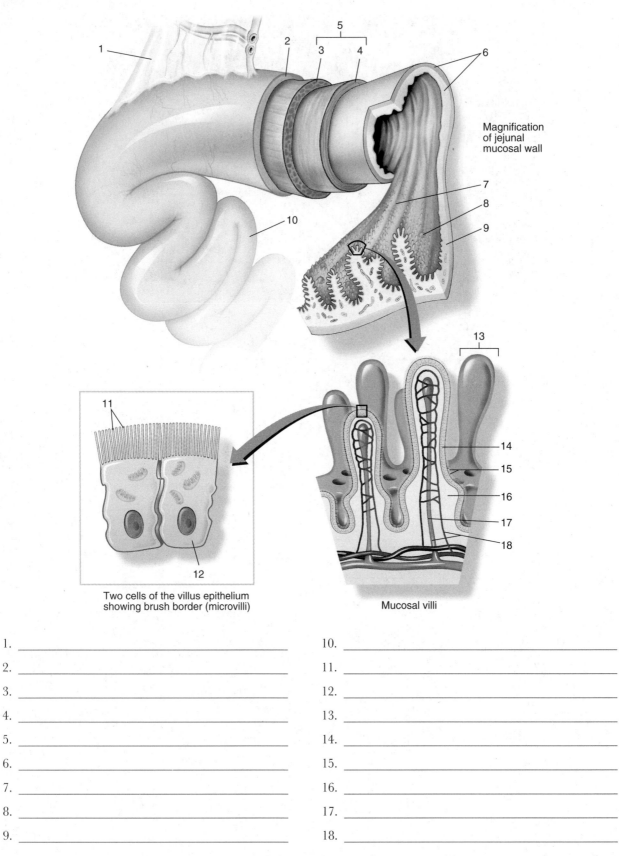

Magnification
of jejunal
mucosal wall

Two cells of the villus epithelium
showing brush border (microvilli)

Mucosal villi

1. _____

2. _____

3. _____

4. _____

5. _____

6. _____

7. _____

8. _____

9. _____

10. _____

11. _____

12. _____

13. _____

14. _____

15. _____

16. _____

17. _____

18. _____

LARGE INTESTINE

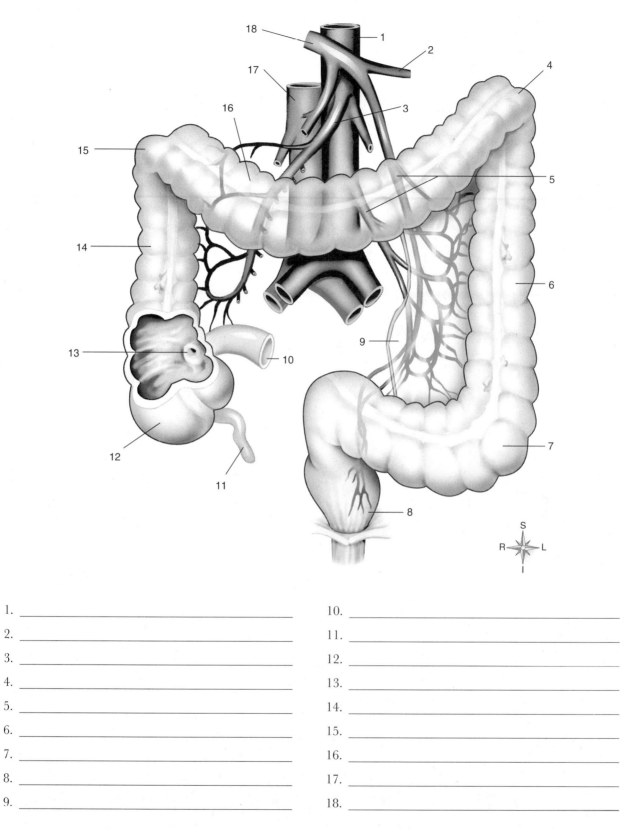

1. _____

2. _____

3. _____

4. _____

5. _____

6. _____

7. _____

8. _____

9. _____

10. _____

11. _____

12. _____

13. _____

14. _____

15. _____

16. _____

17. _____

18. _____

17

Nutrition and Metabolism

Most of us love to eat, but do the foods we enjoy provide us with the basic food types necessary for good nutrition? The body, a finely tuned machine, requires fuel to function properly. A healthy balance of carbohydrates, fats, proteins, vitamins, and minerals is necessary to allow the body to perform at the highest level. These nutrients must be digested, absorbed, and circulated to cells constantly to accommodate the numerous activities that occur throughout the body. The use the body makes of foods once these processes are completed is called *metabolism*.

The liver plays a major role in the metabolism of food. It helps maintain a normal blood glucose level, removes toxins from the blood, processes blood immediately after it leaves the gastrointestinal tract, and initiates the first steps of protein and fat metabolism.

This chapter also discusses basal metabolic rate (BMR). The BMR is the rate at which food is catabolized under basal conditions. This test and the measurement of the amount of protein-bound iodine (PBI) are indirect measures of thyroid gland functioning. The total metabolic rate (TMR) is the amount of energy, expressed in calories, used by the body each day.

Finally, maintaining a constant body temperature is a function of the hypothalamus and a challenge for the metabolic mechanisms of the body. Review of this chapter is necessary to provide you with an understanding of the "fuel" or nutrition necessary to maintain your complex homeostatic machine—the body.

TOPICS FOR REVIEW

Before progressing to Chapter 18, you should be able to define and contrast catabolism and anabolism. Your review should include the metabolic roles of carbohydrates, fats, proteins, vitamins, and minerals. Your study should conclude with an understanding of the basal metabolic rate and physiological mechanisms that regulate body temperature.

METABOLIC FUNCTION OF THE LIVER

Fill in the blanks.

The liver plays an important role in the mechanical digestion of lipids because it secretes (1) _____.
It also produces two of the plasma proteins that play an essential role in blood clotting: (2) _____
and (3) _____. Additionally, liver cells store several substances, notably vitamins A and D and
(4) _____. Finally, the liver is assisted by a unique structural feature of the blood vessels that supply it.
This arrangement, known as the (5) _____ _____ _____, allows toxins to be removed from the
bloodstream before nutrients are distributed throughout the body.

 If you had difficulty with this section, review pages 395-397.

MACRONUTRIENTS AND MICRONUTRIENTS

Match the term with the proper selection.

a. Carbohydrates
b. Fats
c. Proteins
d. Vitamins
e. Minerals

6. _____ Used if cells have inadequate amounts of glucose to catabolize

7. _____ Preferred energy food

8. _____ Amino acids

9. _____ Fat soluble

10. _____ Required for nerve conduction

11. _____ Glycolysis

12. _____ Inorganic elements found naturally in the earth

13. _____ Pyruvic acid

Circle the one that does **not belong.**

14. Glycolysis	Citric acid cycle	ATP	Bile
15. Adipose	Amino acids	Triglycerides	Glycerol
16. A	D	M	K
17. Iron	Proteins	Amino acids	Essential
18. Hydrocortisone	Insulin	Growth hormone	Epinephrine
19. Sodium	Calcium	Zinc	Folic acid
20. Thiamine	Niacin	Ascorbic acid	Riboflavin

➔ *If you had difficulty with this section, review pages 397-401.*

METABOLIC RATES, BODY TEMPERATURE

Select the best answer.

21. The rate at which food is catabolized under basal conditions is the:
    a. TMR
    b. PBI
    c. BMR
    d. ATP

22. The total amount of energy used by the body per day is the:
    a. TMR
    b. PBI
    c. BMR
    d. ATP

23. More than _____ of the energy released from food molecules during catabolism is converted to heat rather than being transferred to ATP.
    a. 20%
    b. 40%
    c. 60%
    d. 80%

24. Maintaining thermoregulation is a function of the:
    a. Thalamus
    b. Hypothalamus
    c. Thyroid
    d. Parathyroids

25. Transfer of heat energy to the skin and then to the external environment is known as:
    a. Radiation
    b. Conduction
    c. Convection
    d. Evaporation

26. A flow of heat waves away from the blood is known as:
    a. Radiation
    b. Conduction
    c. Convection
    d. Evaporation

27. A transfer of heat energy to air that is continually flowing away from the skin is known as:
    a. Radiation
    b. Conduction
    c. Convection
    d. Evaporation

28. Heat absorbed by the process of water vaporization is called:
    a. Radiation
    b. Conduction
    c. Convection
    d. Evaporation

29. A(n) _____ is the amount of energy needed to raise the temperature of 1 gram of water 1° C.
    a. Calorie
    b. Kilocalorie
    c. ATP
    d. BMR

➲ *If you had difficulty with this section, review pages 398 and 401-404.*

UNSCRAMBLE THE WORDS

Unscramble the circled letters and fill in the statement.

30. **L R I E V**

☐ ☐ Ⓞ Ⓞ Ⓞ

31. **T A O B A L I C M S**

☐ Ⓞ Ⓞ ☐ ☐ Ⓞ Ⓞ ☐ ☐ ☐

32. **O M N I A**

Ⓞ ☐ ☐ Ⓞ Ⓞ

33. **Y P U R C V I**

Ⓞ ☐ ☐ ☐ ☐ Ⓞ ☐

How the magician paid his bills.

34.

☐ ☐ ☐ ☐ ☐ ☐ ☐ ☐ ☐ ☐ ☐ ☐

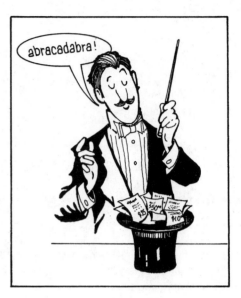

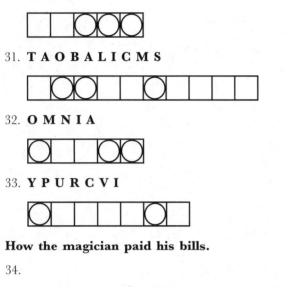

APPLYING WHAT YOU KNOW

35. Dr. Culp was concerned about Deborrah. Her daily food intake provided fewer calories than her TMR. If this trend continues, what will be the result? If it continues over a long period of time, what eating disorder might Deborrah develop?

36. Mrs. Bishop was experiencing fatigue, and a blood test revealed that she was slightly anemic. What mineral will her doctor most likely prescribe? What dietary sources might you suggest that she emphasize in her daily intake?

37. Mrs. Hosmer was training daily for an upcoming marathon. Three days before the 26-mile event, she suddenly quit her daily routine of jogging and switched to a diet high in carbohydrates. Why did Mrs. Hosmer suddenly switch her routine of training?

38. WORD FIND

Can you find 18 terms from this chapter in the box of letters? Words may be spelled top to bottom, bottom to top, right to left, left to right, or diagonally.

```
C  C  C  B  W  E  F  F  L  J  V  G  G  S
A  T  N  L  W  E  U  O  Z  I  E  L  I  B
R  K  K  P  Z  F  R  I  T  P  O  Y  K  L
B  Q  M  I  N  E  R  A  L  S  J  C  C  P
O  S  S  N  C  X  M  I  D  B  D  O  W  P
H  S  I  Y  O  I  T  X  H  I  N  L  S  N
Y  E  L  N  N  I  K  W  W  D  S  Y  N  S
D  G  O  S  O  W  T  I  U  E  H  S  C  N
R  M  B  Y  T  I  W  C  Z  N  N  I  A  A
A  R  A  Q  W  A  T  B  E  I  G  S  J  M
T  E  T  F  N  I  F  A  E  V  E  W  T  Y
E  V  A  P  O  R  A  T  I  O  N  D  T  E
S  I  C  N  E  S  O  P  I  D  A  O  F  E
H  L  Y  K  I  R  E  B  V  P  A  H  C  J
I  W  E  E  P  A  D  F  T  E  A  R  G  G
```

ATP	Conduction	Liver
Adipose	Convection	Minerals
BMR	Evaporation	Proteins
Bile	Fats	Radiation
Carbohydrates	Glycerol	TMR
Catabolism	Glycolysis	Vitamins

❓ DID YOU KNOW?

- Twenty-five years ago, 3%-5% of Americans were deficient in vitamin C. Today, about 15% do not get the amount they need for optimum health.
- The human body has enough fat to produce 7 bars of soap.
- Forty to 50% of body heat can be lost through the head (without a hat) as a result of its extensive circulatory network.

NUTRITION/METABOLISM

Fill in the crossword puzzle.

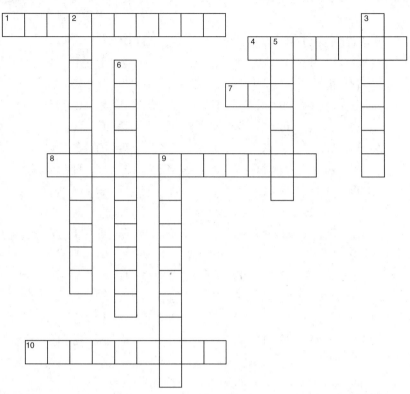

ACROSS

1. Breaks food molecules down, releasing stored energy
4. Amount of energy needed to raise the temperature of 1 gram of water 1° Celsius
7. Rate of metabolism when a person is lying down but awake (abbreviation)
8. A series of reactions that join glucose molecules together to form glycogen
10. Builds food molecules into complex substances

DOWN

2. Occurs when food molecules enter cells and undergo many chemical changes there
3. Organic molecule needed in small quantities for normal metabolism throughout the body
5. Oxygen-using
6. A unit of measure for heat, also known as a large calorie
9. Takes place in the cytoplasm of a cell and changes glucose to pyruvic acid

CHECK YOUR KNOWLEDGE

Multiple Choice

Select the best answer.

1. *Metabolism* is a term that refers to the:
   a. Nutrients that we eat
   b. Use of foods
   c. Building blocks
   d. None of the above

2. Glycolysis changes glucose into:
   a. Pyruvic acid
   b. Carbon dioxide
   c. ATP
   d. None of the above

3. An anaerobic process:
   a. Is an oxygen-using process
   b. Is an oxygen-storing process
   c. Uses no oxygen
   d. Both A and B

4. The amount of nutrients in the blood:
   a. Changes significantly when we exercise
   b. Changes significantly when we go without food for many hours
   c. Does not change very much and remains relatively constant
   d. Both A and B

5. Which of the following hormones lowers blood glucose levels?
   a. Growth hormone
   b. Insulin
   c. Hydrocortisone
   d. Epinephrine

6. Fats not needed for catabolism are anabolized
   to form:
   a. Nonessential amino acids
   b. Triglycerides
   c. Glycogen
   d. ATP

7. Essential amino acids:
   a. Must be in the diet
   b. Can be made by the body
   c. Make up the majority of the 20 amino acids
   d. All of the above

8. A good source of iron in the diet is:
   a. Meat
   b. Dairy products
   c. Seafood
   d. Fruits

9. The flow of heat waves away from the blood is known as:
   a. Conduction
   b. Radiation
   c. Convection
   d. Evaporation

10. The liver:
    a. Plays an important role in the mechanical digestion of lipids because it secretes bile
    b. Detoxifies various poisonous substances such as bacterial products and certain drugs
    c. Synthesizes several kinds of protein compounds
    d. All of the above

Fill in the blanks.

11. The preferred energy food of the body is _____.

12. An anaerobic process is _____.

13. An aerobic process is the _____ _____ _____.

14. A deficiency of _____ may result in a goiter.

15. The rate at which food is catabolized under basal conditions is known as the _____ _____ _____.

16. The total amount of energy used by the body per day is the _____ _____ _____.

17. Maintaining homeostasis of temperature is the function of the _____.

18. All the chemical reactions that release energy from food molecules make up the process of _____.

19. The many chemical reactions that build food molecules into more complex chemical compounds constitute the process of _____.

20. Four fat-soluble vitamins that can be stored in the liver for later use are _____, _____, _____, and _____.

CHAPTER 18

Urinary System

Living produces wastes. Wherever people live or work or play, wastes accumulate. To keep these areas healthy, there must be a method—such as a sanitation department—of disposing of these wastes.

Wastes accumulate in your body also. The conversion of food and gases into substances and energy necessary for survival results in waste products. A large percentage of these wastes is removed by the urinary system.

Two vital organs, the kidneys, cleanse the blood of the many waste products that are continually produced as a result of the metabolism of food in the body cells. They eliminate these wastes in the form of urine.

Urine formation is the result of three processes: filtration, reabsorption, and secretion. These processes occur in successive portions of the microscopic units of the kidneys known as *nephrons*. The amount of urine produced by the nephrons is controlled primarily by the hormones ADH and aldosterone.

After urine is produced it is drained from the renal pelvis by the ureters to flow into the bladder. The bladder then stores the urine until it is voided through the urethra.

If waste products are allowed to accumulate in the body, they soon become poisonous, a condition called *uremia*. Knowledge of the urinary system is necessary to understand how the body rids itself of waste and avoids toxicity.

TOPICS FOR REVIEW

Before progressing to Chapter 19 you should have an understanding of the structure and function of the organs of the urinary system. Your review should include knowledge of the nephron and its role in urine production. Your study should conclude with a review of the three main processes involved in urine production and the mechanisms that control urine volume.

KIDNEYS—FORMATION OF URINE—CONTROL OF URINE VOLUME

Multiple Choice

Select the best answer.

1. The outermost portion of the kidney is known as the:
   a. Medulla
   b. Papilla
   c. Pelvis
   d. Pyramid
   e. Cortex

2. The saclike structure that surrounds the glomerulus is the:
   a. Renal pelvis
   b. Calyx
   c. Bowman capsule
   d. Cortex
   e. None of the above

3. The renal corpuscle is made up of the:
   a. Bowman capsule and proximal convoluted tubule
   b. Glomerulus and proximal convoluted tubule
   c. Bowman capsule and distal convoluted tubule
   d. Glomerulus and distal convoluted tubule
   e. Bowman capsule and glomerulus

4. Which of the following functions is *not* performed by the kidneys?
   a. Maintenance of homeostasis
   b. Removal of wastes from the blood
   c. Production of ADH
   d. Removal of electrolytes from the blood

5. _____ percent of the glomerular filtrate is reabsorbed.
   a. Twenty
   b. Forty
   c. Seventy-five
   d. Eighty-five
   e. Ninety-nine

6. The glomerular filtration rate is _____ mL per minute.
   a. 1.25
   b. 12.5
   c. 125.0
   d. 1250.0
   e. None of the above

7. Glucose is reabsorbed in the:
   a. Henle loop
   b. Proximal convoluted tubule
   c. Distal convoluted tubule
   d. Glomerulus
   e. None of the above

8. Reabsorption does *not* occur in the:
   a. Nephron loop
   b. Proximal convoluted tubule
   c. Distal convoluted tubule
   d. Collecting duct
   e. Calyx

9. The greater the amount of salt intake, the:
   a. Less salt excreted in the urine
   b. More salt reabsorbed
   c. More salt excreted in the urine
   d. None of the above

10. Which one of the following substances is secreted by diffusion?
    a. Sodium ions
    b. Certain drugs
    c. Ammonia
    d. Hydrogen ions
    e. Potassium ions

11. Which of the following statements about ADH is *not* true?
    a. It is stored by the pituitary gland.
    b. It makes the collecting tubules less permeable to water.
    c. It makes the distal convoluted tubules more permeable.
    d. It is produced by the hypothalamus.

12. Which of the following statements about aldosterone is *not* true?
    a. It is secreted by the adrenal cortex.
    b. It is a water-retaining hormone.
    c. It is a salt-retaining hormone.
    d. All of the above are correct.

➜ *If you had difficulty with this section, review pages 408-419.*

Matching

Choose the correct term and write the letter in the space next to the appropriate definition below.

a. Medulla
b. Cortex
c. Pyramids
d. Papilla
e. Pelvis
f. Calyx
g. Nephrons

h. Uremia
i. Proteinuria
j. Bowman capsule
k. Glomerulus
l. Nephron loop
m. Juxtaglomerular apparatus
n. Glycosuria

13. _____ Functioning unit of urinary system

14. _____ Abnormally large amounts of plasma proteins in the urine

15. _____ Uremic poisoning

16. _____ Outer part of kidney

17. _____ Together with the Bowman capsule forms renal corpuscle

18. _____ Division of the renal pelvis

19. _____ Cup-shaped top of a nephron

20. _____ Innermost end of a pyramid

21. _____ Extension of proximal tubule

22. _____ Triangular-shaped divisions of the medulla of the kidney

23. _____ Functions in blood volume and blood pressure regulation

24. _____ Inner portion of kidney

➡ *If you had difficulty with this section, review pages 411-414 and 423.*

ELIMINATION OF URINE—URETERS, URINARY BLADDER, AND URETHRA

Indicate which organ is identified by the following descriptions by writing the appropriate letter in the answer blank.

a. Ureters
b. Bladder
c. Urethra

25. _____ Rugae

26. _____ Lowermost part of urinary tract

27. _____ Lining membrane richly supplied with sensory nerve endings

28. _____ Lies behind pubic symphysis

29. _____ Dual function in male

30. _____ 1½ inches long in female

31. _____ Drains renal pelvis

32. _____ Surrounded by prostate in male

33. _____ Elastic fibers and involuntary muscle fibers

34. _____ 10-12 inches long

35. _____ Trigone

Fill in the blanks.

36. _____ _____ is the description of the pain caused by the passage of a kidney stone.

37. The urinary tract is lined with _____ _____.

38. Another name for kidney stones is _____ _____.

39. A technique that uses _____ to pulverize stones, thus avoiding surgery, is being used to treat kidney stones.

40. Older people generally have a lower overall lean body mass and, therefore, a(n) _____ production of waste products that must be excreted from the body.

41. The _____ _____ is the basinlike upper end of the ureter located inside the kidney.

42. In the male, the urethra serves as a passageway for both urine and _____.

43. The external opening of the urethra is the _____ _____.

➡ *If you had difficulty with this section, review pages 419-421.*

MICTURITION—URINALYSIS

Fill in the blanks.

The terms (44) _____, (45) _____, and (46) _____ all refer to the passage of urine from the body or the emptying of the bladder. The sphincters guard the bladder. The (47) _____ _____ sphincter is located at the bladder (48) _____ and is involuntary. The external urethral sphincter is formed of (49) _____ muscle and is under (50) _____ control.

As the bladder fills, nervous impulses are transmitted to the spinal cord and a(n) (51) _____ _____ is initiated. Urine then enters the (52) _____ to be eliminated.

Urinary (53) _____ is a condition in which no urine is voided. Urinary (54) _____ is when the kidneys do not produce any urine, but the bladder retains its ability to empty itself. The term (55) _____ _____ refers to urine loss associated with laughing, coughing, or heavy lifting.

In clinical and laboratory situations a standard urinalysis is often referred to as a (56) _____ and (57) _____ urinalysis. Changes in the normal characteristics of urine may be a sign of (58) _____.

➡ *If you had difficulty with this section, review pages 421-423.*

UNSCRAMBLE THE WORDS

Unscramble the circled letters and fill in the statement.

59. **A Y X L C**

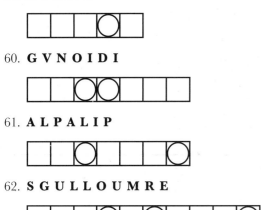

			◯	

60. **G V N O I D I**

		◯	◯			

61. **A L P A L I P**

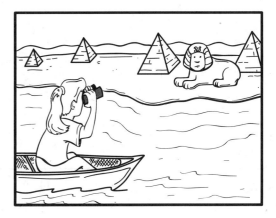

		◯			◯

62. **S G U L L O U M R E**

			◯		◯			◯

What Betty saw while cruising down the Nile.

63.

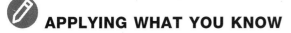

✎ APPLYING WHAT YOU KNOW

64. John suffered from low levels of ADH. What primary urinary symptom would he notice?

65. Bud was in a diving accident and his spinal cord was severed. He was paralyzed from the waist down and as a result was incontinent. His physician was concerned about the continuous residual urine buildup. What was the reason for concern?

66. Caryl had a prolonged surgical procedure and experienced problems with urinary retention postoperatively. A urinary catheter was inserted into her bladder for the elimination of urine. Several days later Caryl developed cystitis. What might be a possible cause?

67. WORD FIND

Can you find 18 terms from the chapter in the box of letters? Words may be spelled top to bottom, bottom to top, right to left, left to right, or diagonally.

```
H N O I T I R U T C I M N M Y
V E Q N G A L L I P A P S E S
T P M C O L D U J Y S I N D D
L H G O X I O W C G V D I U J
C R F N D B T M T L I M B K L
P O O T X I C A E K A P X L D
Q N U I E G A P R R T C W A O
B J R N T T L L Y T U Y G D M
S D E E R G Y P Y V L L P H Z
I H T N O U X W D S X I U J G
M X E C C Y S T I T I S F S Q
J O R E D D A L B U E S G B S
Y I S E B V L L B H V Q L U L
```

ADH	Filtration	Micturition
Bladder	Glomerulus	Nephron
Calculi	Hemodialysis	Papilla
Calyx	Incontinence	Pelvis
Cortex	Kidney	Pyramids
Cystitis	Medulla	Ureters

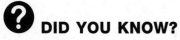 **DID YOU KNOW?**

- If the tubules in a kidney were stretched out and untangled, there would be 70 miles of them.
- While examining urine, German chemist Hennig Brand discovered phosphorus.
- People adrift at sea or lost in the desert for long periods often resort to drinking their urine when no rainwater is available. This, however, will not prevent you from dying of dehydration, especially if it causes vomiting.

URINARY SYSTEM

Fill in the crossword puzzle.

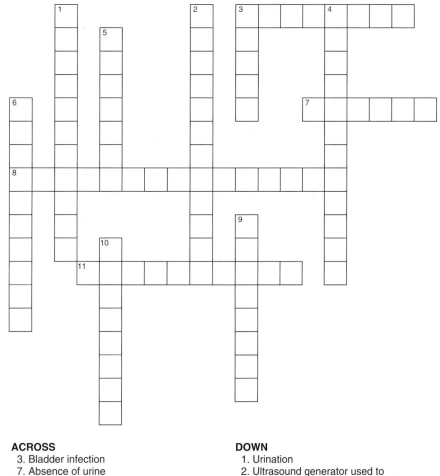

ACROSS
3. Bladder infection
7. Absence of urine
8. Passage of a tube into the bladder to withdraw urine
11. Network of blood capillaries tucked into Bowman capsule

DOWN
1. Urination
2. Ultrasound generator used to break up kidney stones
3. Division of the renal pelvis
4. Voiding involuntarily
5. Area on posterior bladder wall free of rugae
6. Glucose in the urine
9. Large amount of urine
10. Scanty urine

CHECK YOUR KNOWLEDGE

Multiple Choice

Select the best answer.

1. Which of the following is *not* true of the kidneys?
   a. The right kidney is lower than the left.
   b. They are retroperitoneal.
   c. The rate of blood flow through the kidneys is among the highest in the body.
   d. All of the above are true.

2. The Bowman capsule and the glomerulus make up the:
   a. Renal tubule
   b. Renal corpuscle
   c. Nephron loop
   d. Collecting tubule

3. The kidneys serve the body by:
   a. Maintaining homeostasis
   b. Excreting toxins and waste products containing nitrogen
   c. Regulating the proper balance between body water content and salt
   d. All of the above

4. Urine formation begins with:
   a. Glomerular filtration
   b. The proximal convoluted tubule
   c. The distal convoluted tubule
   d. Henle loop

5. A well-known sign of diabetes mellitus is:
   a. Proteinuria
   b. Oliguria
   c. Glycosuria
   d. Anuria

6. A lithotriptor is used for:
   a. Diabetes mellitus
   b. Incontinence
   c. Renal calculi
   d. Oliguria

7. Aldosterone:
   a. Assists in controlling the kidney tubules' excretion of salt
   b. Stimulates the tubules to reabsorb sodium salts at a faster rate
   c. Decreases tubular water reabsorption
   d. Is a salt- and water-losing hormone

8. Control of urine volume is maintained primarily by the:
   a. Bowman capsule
   b. Nephron loop
   c. ADH from the posterior pituitary gland
   d. Kidney tubule

9. Which is *not* a part of the kidney?
   a. Cortex
   b. Trigone
   c. Medulla
   d. Pyramids

10. Which of the following is *not* a primary process in urine formation?
    a. Active transport
    b. Filtration
    c. Reabsorption
    d. Secretion

Matching

Select the most correct answer from column B for each statement in column A. (Only one answer is correct.)

Column A

11. _____ Uremia

12. _____ Nephrons

13. _____ Renal tubule

14. _____ Juxtaglomerular apparatus

15. _____ Secretion

16. _____ CAPD

17. _____ Cystitis

18. _____ Emptying reflex

19. _____ Calyces

20. _____ Pyramids

Column B

a. Urinary bladder infection
b. Triangular divisions of medulla of kidney
c. Microscopic units of kidney
d. Blood pressure regulation
e. Uremic poisoning
f. Nephron loop
g. Relaxation of internal sphincter
h. Renal failure
i. Divisions of renal pelvis
j. Hydrogen and potassium ions

URINARY SYSTEM

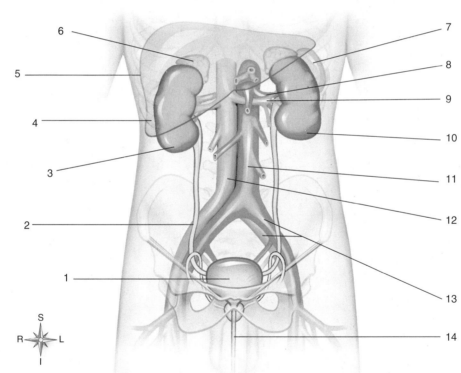

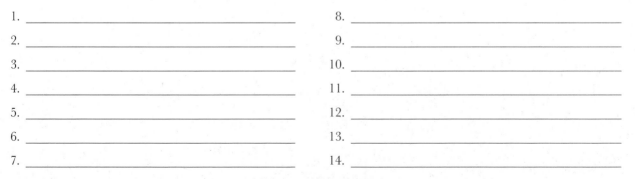

1. _____

2. _____

3. _____

4. _____

5. _____

6. _____

7. _____

8. _____

9. _____

10. _____

11. _____

12. _____

13. _____

14. _____

KIDNEY

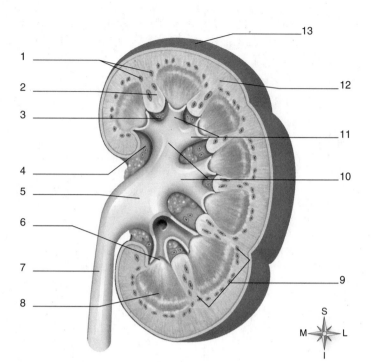

1. _____
2. _____
3. _____
4. _____
5. _____
6. _____
7. _____

8. _____
9. _____
10. _____
11. _____
12. _____
13. _____

NEPHRON

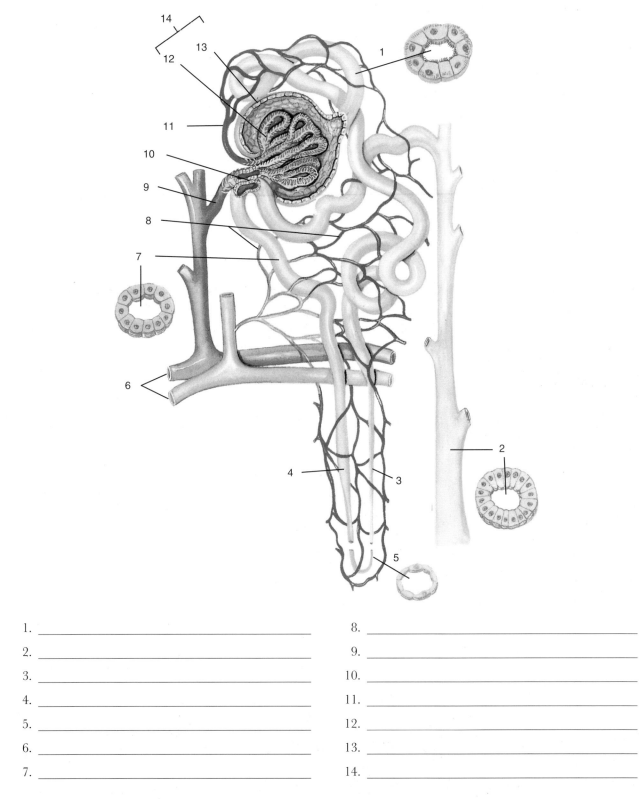

1. _____
2. _____
3. _____
4. _____
5. _____
6. _____
7. _____
8. _____
9. _____
10. _____
11. _____
12. _____
13. _____
14. _____

CHAPTER 19
Fluid and Electrolyte Balance

In the very first chapter of the text, you learned that survival depends on the body's ability to maintain or restore homeostasis. Specifically, *homeostasis* means that the body fluids remain constant within very narrow limits. These fluids are classified as either intracellular fluid (ICF) or extracellular fluid (ECF). As the names imply, intracellular fluid lies within the cells and extracellular fluid is located outside the cells. A balance between these two fluids is maintained by certain body mechanisms: (a) the adjustment of fluid output to fluid intake under normal circumstances; (b) the concentration of electrolytes in the extracellular fluid; (c) the capillary blood pressure; and (d) the concentration of proteins in the blood.

Comprehension of how these mechanisms maintain and restore fluid balance is necessary for an understanding of the complexities of homeostasis and its relationship to the survival of the individual.

TOPICS FOR REVIEW

Before progressing to Chapter 20, you should review the types of body fluids and their subdivisions. Your study should include the mechanisms that maintain fluid balance and the nature and importance of electrolytes in body fluids. You should be able to give examples of common fluid imbalances and have an understanding of the role of fluid and electrolyte balance in the maintenance of homeostasis.

BODY FLUID VOLUMES AND COMPARTMENTS

Circle the correct answer.

1. The largest volume of body fluid by far lies (*inside* or *outside*) cells.

2. Interstitial fluid is (*intracellular* or *extracellular*).

3. Plasma is (*intracellular* or *extracellular*).

4. Obese people have a (*lower* or *higher*) water content per pound of body weight than thin people.

5. Infants have (*more* or *less*) water in comparison to body weight than adults of either sex.

6. There is a rapid (*increase* or *decline*) in the proportion of body water to body weight during the first 10 years of life.

7. The female body contains slightly (*more* or *less*) water per pound of weight.

8. In general, as age increases, the amount of water per pound of body weight (*increases* or *decreases*).

9. Excluding adipose tissue, approximately (*55%* or *85%*) of body weight is water.

10. The term (*fluid balance* or *fluid compartments*) means the volumes of ICF, IF, plasma, and the total volume of water in the body all remain relatively constant.

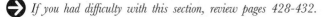 *If you had difficulty with this section, review pages 428-432.*

MECHANISMS THAT MAINTAIN FLUID BALANCE

Multiple Choice

Select the best answer.

11. Which one of the following is a positively charged ion?
    a. Sodium
    b. Chloride
    c. Phosphate
    d. Bicarbonate

12. Which one of the following is a negatively charged ion?
    a. Sodium
    b. Potassium
    c. Calcium
    d. Chloride

13. If the blood sodium concentration increases, then blood volume will:
    a. Increase
    b. Decrease
    c. Remain the same
    d. None of the above

14. The smallest amount of water comes from:
    a. Water in foods that are eaten
    b. Ingested liquids
    c. Water formed from catabolism
    d. None of the above

15. The greatest amount of water lost from the body is from the:
    a. Lungs
    b. Skin, by diffusion
    c. Skin, by sweat
    d. Feces
    e. Kidneys

16. Which one of the following is the most important factor in determining urine volume?
    a. The concentration of electrolytes in the extracellular fluid
    b. The capillary blood pressure
    c. The concentration of proteins in blood
    d. The rate of water and salt reabsorption from the renal tubules

17. The type of fluid output that changes the most is:
    a. Water loss in the feces
    b. Water loss across the skin
    c. Water loss via the lungs
    d. Water loss in the urine
    e. None of the above

18. Which of the following is *not* correct?
    a. Fluid output must equal fluid intake.
    b. ADH controls salt reabsorption in the kidney.
    c. Water follows sodium.
    d. Renal tubule regulation of salt and water is the most important factor in determining urine volume.

19. Diuretics work on all of the following *except* the:
    a. Proximal tubule
    b. Henle loop
    c. Distal tubule
    d. Collecting ducts
    e. Diuretics work on all of the above

20. Of all the sodium-containing secretions, the one with the largest volume is:
    a. Saliva
    b. Gastric secretions
    c. Bile
    d. Pancreatic juice
    e. Intestinal secretions

21. The higher the capillary blood pressure, the _____ the amount of interstitial fluid.
    a. Smaller
    b. Larger
    c. There is no relationship between capillary blood pressure and volume of interstitial fluid.

22. An increase in capillary blood pressure will lead to _____ in blood volume.
    a. An increase
    b. A decrease
    c. No change
    d. None of the above

23. Which one of the fluid compartments varies the most in volume?
    a. Intracellular
    b. Interstitial
    c. Extracellular
    d. Plasma

24. Which one of the following will *not* cause edema?
    a. The retention of electrolytes in the interstitial fluid
    b. An increase in capillary blood pressure
    c. Burns
    d. A decrease in the concentration of plasma proteins
    e. All of the above may cause edema

True or False

If the statement is true, write "T" in the answer blank. If the statement is false, correct the statement by circling the incorrect term and writing the correct term in the answer blank.

25. _____ The three sources of fluid intake are the liquids we drink, the foods we eat, and the water formed by the anabolism of foods.

26. _____ The body maintains fluid balance mainly by changing the volume of urine excreted to match changes in the volume of fluid intake.

27. _____ Some output of fluid will occur as long as life continues.

28. _____ Glucose is an example of an electrolyte.

29. _____ Excess aldosterone leads to hypovolemia.

30. _____ Typical daily intake and output totals should be approximately 1,200 mL.

31. _____ Bile is a sodium-containing internal secretion.

32. _____ The average daily diet contains about 500 mEq of sodium.

FLUID IMBALANCES

Fill in the blanks.

(33) _____ is the fluid imbalance seen most often. In this condition, interstitial fluid volume (34) _____ first, but eventually, if treatment has not been given, intracellular fluid and plasma volumes (35) _____. (36) _____ can also occur, but is much less common.

Giving (37) _____ _____ too rapidly or in too large amounts can put too heavy a burden on the (38) _____.

 If you had difficulty with this section, review pages 432-438.

ELECTROLYTE IMBALANCES

Fill in the blanks.

39. Hyponatremia occurs when there is relatively too much _____ in the ECF compartment for the amount of sodium present.

40. _____ is the clinical term used to describe blood potassium levels of more than 5.1 mEq/L.

41. _____ is the most abundant mineral in the body.

42. _____ occurs when blood calcium levels rise above normal limits.

 If you had difficulty with this section, review pages 437-440.

UNSCRAMBLE THE WORDS

Unscramble the circled letters and fill in the statement.

43. **M D E E A**

44. **D F I L U**

45. **N I O**

46. **S O U I T N V A R E N**

What Gary's dad disliked most about his music.

47.

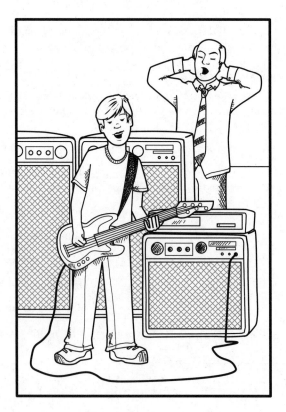

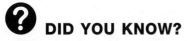

APPLYING WHAT YOU KNOW

48. Mrs. Titus was asked to keep an accurate record of her fluid intake and output. She was concerned because the two did not balance. What is a possible explanation for this?

49. Nurse Briker was caring for a patient who was receiving diuretics. What special nursing implications should be followed for patients on this therapy?

50. WORD FIND

Can you find the 12 terms from this chapter in the box of letters? Words may be spelled top to bottom, bottom to top, right to left, left to right, or diagonally.

```
S T V H O M E O S T A S I S H
I E D E M A S Q A L P U E G L
M M L U F L U I D O Y O I S L
W S B E A E C O L D P N I E R
L I T A C V S H Q O C E H B C
L L X J L T E A W Y B V Q Q O
I O O P E A R U C T C A A R I
N B H R X S N O I I P R T C N
S A O X M G J C L N J T B A H
I N X X D V U D E Y K N Y O C
E A A J Q D I U R E T I C S X
I F C J A M P V E N B E Y F W
V F K T Q X R M D D S I V O T
E T T Z N T R P X I M L J F I
S W Y A P V Q N S K T K W B P
```

Aldosterone	Edema	Imbalance
Anabolism	Electrolyte	Intravenous
Catabolism	Fluid	Ions
Diuretics	Homeostasis	Kidney

DID YOU KNOW?

- The best fluid replacement drink is 1/4 teaspoon of table salt to 1 quart of water.
- If all of the water were drained from the body of an average 160-pound man, the body would weigh 64 pounds.
- The average person can live up to 11 days without water, assuming a mean environmental temperature of 60° F.

FLUID/ELECTROLYTES

Fill in the crossword puzzle.

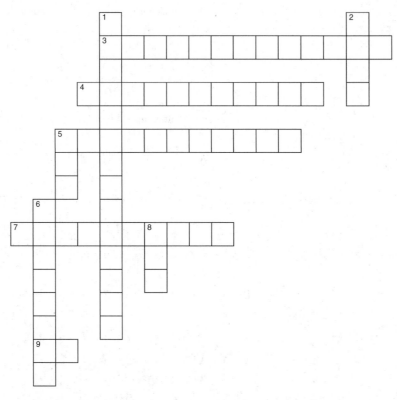

ACROSS
3. Result of rapidly given intravenous fluids
4. Result of large loss of body fluids
5. Compound that dissociates in solution into ions
7. To break up
9. A subdivision of extracellular fluid (abbreviation)

DOWN
1. Organic substance that doesn't dissociate in solution
2. Dissociated particles of an electrolyte that carry an electrical charge
5. Fluid outside cells (abbreviation)
6. "Causing urine"
8. Fluid inside cells (abbreviation)

CHECK YOUR KNOWLEDGE

Multiple Choice

Select the best answer.

1. Which of the following have the most water compared with body weight?
   a. Infants
   b. Females
   c. Males
   d. All of the above have the same percentage of water to body weight.

2. Which of the following acts as a mechanism for controlling plasma, IF, and ICF volumes?
   a. The concentration of electrolytes in ECF
   b. The capillary blood pressure
   c. The concentration of proteins in blood
   d. All of the above

3. Which of the following statements is true regarding maintenance of fluid homeostasis?
   a. The type of fluid output that changes most is urine volume.
   b. Renal tubule regulation of salt and water is the most important factor in determining urine volume.
   c. The presence of sodium causes water to move.
   d. All of the above are true.

4. Which of the following is *not* a normal portal of exit for water from the body?
   a. Diffusion
   b. Lungs
   c. Water formed by catabolism
   d. Intestines

5. The fluid imbalance that is seen most often is:
   a. Dehydration
   b. Increased plasma volumes
   c. Overhydration
   d. Sunstroke

6. Congestive heart failure is the most common cause of:
   a. Overhydration
   b. Edema
   c. Dehydration
   d. Decreased capillary hydrostatic pressure

7. The kidney acts as the chief regulator of:
   a. Aldosterone
   b. Ingested liquids
   c. Perspiration
   d. Sodium in body fluids

8. Excess aldosterone leads to:
   a. Hypervolemia
   b. Hypovolemia
   c. Hypertension
   d. Hypotension

9. Which of the following is the most abundant body fluid in a young adult male?
   a. Intracellular fluid
   b. Interstitial fluid
   c. Plasma
   d. Blood

10. The average ingested liquid intake per day is:
    a. 500 mL
    b. 750 mL
    c. 1,000 mL
    d. 1,500 mL

Matching

Select the most correct answer from column B for each statement in column A. (Only one answer is correct.)

Column A

11. _____ Extracellular

12. _____ Intracellular

13. _____ Nonelectrolyte

14. _____ Electrolyte

15. _____ Diuretic

16. _____ Fluid balance

17. _____ Edema

18. _____ Prolonged diarrhea

19. _____ Rapid IV fluids

20. _____ Hypothalamus

21. _____ Capillary blood pressure

22. _____ ANH

23. _____ Anions

24. _____ Pitting edema

25. _____ Cations

Column B

a. Glucose

b. Inside cells

c. Homeostasis

d. Stimulates production of urine

e. Plasma

f. Fluid imbalance

g. Dehydration

h. Overhydration

i. "Water-pushing" force

j. Table salt

k. Positively charged ions

l. Hormone

m. Negatively charged ions

n. Subcutaneous swelling in ankles and feet

o. Thirst centers

CHAPTER 20
Acid-Base Balance

It has been established in previous chapters that an equilibrium between intracellular and extracellular fluid volume must exist for homeostasis to be maintained. Equally important to homeostasis is the chemical acid-base balance of the body fluids. The degree of acidity or alkalinity of a body fluid is expressed in pH value. The neutral point, where a fluid would be neither acid nor alkaline, is pH 7. Increasing acidity is expressed as less than 7, and increasing alkalinity is expressed as greater than 7. Examples of body fluids that are acidic are gastric juice (1.6) and urine (6.0). Blood, on the other hand, is considered alkaline with a pH of 7.45.

Buffers are substances that prevent a sharp change in the pH of a fluid when an acid or base is added to it. They are one of several mechanisms that are constantly monitoring the pH of fluids in the body. If, for any reason, these mechanisms do not function properly, a pH imbalance occurs. These two kinds of imbalances are known as *alkalosis* and *acidosis*.

Maintaining the acid-base balance of body fluids is a matter of vital importance. If this balance varies even slightly, necessary chemical and cellular reactions cannot occur. Your review of this chapter is necessary to understand the delicate acid-base balance necessary to survival.

TOPICS FOR REVIEW

Before progressing to Chapter 21, you should have an understanding of the pH of body fluids and the mechanisms that control the pH of these fluids in the body. Your study should conclude with a review of the metabolic and respiratory types of pH imbalances.

pH OF BODY FLUIDS

Choose the correct term from the options given and write the letter in the answer blank.

a. Acid
b. Base

1. _____ Lower concentration of hydrogen ions than hydroxide ions

2. _____ Higher concentration of hydrogen ions than hydroxide ions

3. _____ Gastric juice

4. _____ Saliva

5. _____ Arterial blood

6. _____ Venous blood

7. _____ Apple juice

8. _____ Milk

9. _____ Ammonia

10. _____ Pancreatic fluid

→ *If you had difficulty with this section, review pages 444-447.*

MECHANISMS THAT CONTROL pH OF BODY FLUIDS—pH IMBALANCES

Multiple Choice

Select the best answer.

11. When carbon dioxide enters the blood, it reacts with the enzyme carbonic anhydrase to form:
    a. Sodium bicarbonate
    b. Water and carbon dioxide
    c. Ammonium chloride
    d. Bicarbonate ion
    e. Carbonic acid

12. The lungs remove _____ liters of carbonic acid each day.
    a. 10
    b. 15
    c. 20
    d. 25
    e. 30

13. When a buffer reacts with a strong acid, it changes the strong acid to a:
    a. Weak acid
    b. Strong base
    c. Weak base
    d. Water
    e. None of the above

14. Which one of the following is *not* a change in the blood that results from the buffering of fixed acids in tissue capillaries?
    a. The amount of carbonic acid increases slightly.
    b. The amount of bicarbonate in blood decreases.
    c. The hydrogen ion concentration of blood increases slightly.
    d. The blood pH decreases slightly.
    e. All of the above are changes that result from the buffering of fixed acids in tissue capillaries.

15. The most abundant acid in the body is:
    a. HCl
    b. Lactic acid
    c. Carbonic acid
    d. Acetic acid
    e. Sulfuric acid

16. The normal ratio of sodium bicarbonate to carbonic acid in arterial blood is:
    a. 5:1
    b. 10:1
    c. 15:1
    d. 20:1
    e. None of the above

17. Which of the following would *not* be a consequence of holding your breath?
    a. The amount of carbonic acid in the blood increases.
    b. The blood pH decreases.
    c. The body develops an alkalosis.
    d. No carbon dioxide leaves the body.

18. Which of the following is *not* true of the kidneys?
    a. They can eliminate larger amounts of acid than the lungs.
    b. More bases than acids are usually excreted by the kidneys.
    c. If the kidneys fail, homeostasis of acid-base balance fails.
    d. They are the most effective regulators of blood pH.

19. The pH of the urine may be as low as:
    a. 1.6
    b. 2.5
    c. 3.2
    d. 4.8
    e. 7.4

20. In the distal tubule cells, the product of the reaction aided by carbonic anhydrase is:
    a. Water
    b. Carbon dioxide
    c. Water and carbon dioxide
    d. Hydrogen ions
    e. Carbonic acid

True or False

If the statement is true, write "T" in the answer blank. If the statement is false, correct the statement by circling the incorrect term and writing the correct term in the answer blank.

21. _____ Any factor that causes an appreciable decrease in respirations may, in time, cause alkalosis.

22. _____ The body has three mechanisms for regulating the pH of its fluids. They are the heart mechanism, the respiratory mechanism, and the urinary mechanism.

23. _____ Buffers consist of two kinds of substances and are, therefore, often called duobuffers.

24. _____ Ordinary baking soda is one of the main buffers of the normally occurring "fixed" acids in the blood.

25. _____ The accumulation of ketone bodies in the blood results from excessive metabolism of fats most often seen in uncontrolled type 1 diabetes.

26. _____ Anything that causes an excessive increase in respirations will in time produce acidosis.

27. _____ The lungs are the body's most effective regulator of blood pH.

28. _____ More acids than bases are usually excreted by the kidneys because more acids than bases usually enter the blood.

29. _____ Blood levels of sodium bicarbonate can be regulated by the lungs.

30. _____ Blood levels of carbonic acid can be regulated by the kidneys.

➡ *If you had difficulty with this section, review pages 447-450.*

pH IMBALANCES—METABOLIC AND RESPIRATORY DISTURBANCES—COMPENSATION FOR pH IMBALANCES

Write the letter of the correct term on the blank next to the appropriate definition.

31. _____ Emesis

32. _____ Uncontrolled type 1 diabetes

33. _____ Chloride-containing solution

34. _____ Bicarbonate deficit

35. _____ Present during emesis

36. _____ Bicarbonate excess

37. _____ Rapid breathing

38. _____ Carbonic acid excess

39. _____ Carbonic acid deficit

40. _____ Hyperventilation syndrome

a. Metabolic acidosis
b. Metabolic alkalosis
c. Respiratory acidosis
d. Respiratory alkalosis
e. Vomiting
f. Normal saline
g. Ketoacidosis
h. Hyperventilation
i. Hypersalivation
j. Anxiety

➔ *If you had difficulty with this section, review pages 450-454.*

UNSCRAMBLE THE WORDS

Unscramble the circled letters and fill in the statement.

41. **U L I F D S**

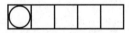

42. **E B T I A C N A O B R**

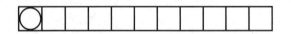

43. **A B S E**

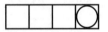

44. **X F D E I**

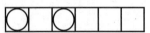

45. **R O G H Y N E D**

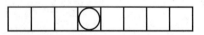

How Sam the "stunt man" used his mattress.

46.

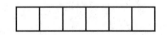

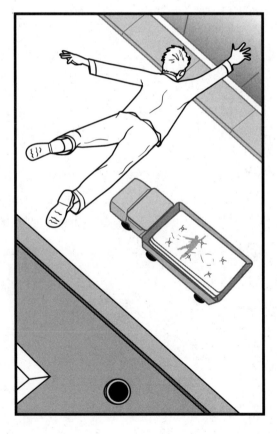

✎ **APPLYING WHAT YOU KNOW**

47. Holly was pregnant and was experiencing repeated vomiting episodes for several days. Her doctor became concerned, admitted her to the hospital, and began intravenous administration of normal saline. How will this help Holly?

48. Cara had a minor bladder infection. She had heard that this is often the result of the urine being less acidic than necessary and that she should drink cranberry juice to correct the acid problem. She had no cranberry juice, so she decided to substitute orange juice. What was wrong with this substitution?

49. Mr. Almaguer has frequent bouts of hyperacidity of the stomach. Which will assist in neutralizing the acid more promptly: milk or Milk of Magnesia?

50. WORD FIND

Can you find 18 terms from this chapter in the box of letters? Words may be spelled top to bottom, bottom to top, right to left, left to right, or diagonally.

```
S  I  S  A  T  S  O  E  M  O  H  P  R  G
E  C  N  A  L  A  B  D  I  U  L  F  E  F
T  S  Y  E  N  D  I  K  W  T  I  K  A  J
Y  D  M  N  D  E  J  W  L  P  T  D  J  I
L  D  N  O  L  H  V  W  O  U  H  D  O  I
O  V  E  R  H  Y  D  R  A  T  I  O  N  S
R  E  I  E  E  D  E  M  A  U  R  O  R  Q
T  L  M  T  C  R  U  L  R  F  S  E  O  Y
C  C  U  S  Z  A  W  E  K  A  T  N  I  X
E  O  Z  O  T  T  A  N  A  U  N  M  F
L  F  K  D  P  I  O  I  W  W  Q  L  G  Q
E  N  I  L  C  O  O  H  O  W  S  B  X  S
N  J  X  A  L  N  F  S  U  N  L  J  J  J
O  C  U  V  S  A  L  G  T  I  S  C  Z  X
N  I  Z  L  L  D  Y  X  Q  Q  K  D  C  D
```

ADH	Edema	Nonelectrolytes
Aldosterone	Electrolytes	Output
Anions	Fluid balance	Overhydration
Cations	Homeostasis	Sodium
Dehydration	Intake	Thirst
Diuretic	Kidneys	Water

❓ DID YOU KNOW?

- The brain is a 3-pound greedy organ that demands 17% of all cardiac output and 20% of all available oxygen.
- English ships carried limes to protect the sailors from scurvy. American ships carried cranberries.
- Arterial blood gas (ABG) measurement will give the information needed to determine if the primary disturbance of acid-base balance is respiratory or metabolic in nature.

ACID/BASE BALANCE

Fill in the crossword puzzle.

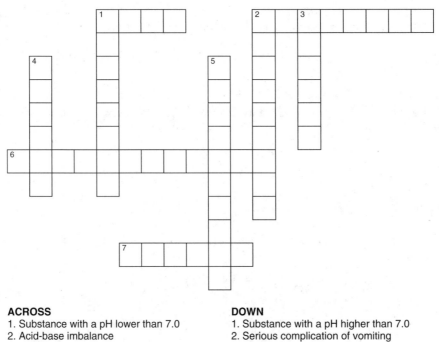

ACROSS
1. Substance with a pH lower than 7.0
2. Acid-base imbalance
6. Results from the excessive metabolism of fats in uncontrolled diabetics (2 words)
7. Vomitus

DOWN
1. Substance with a pH higher than 7.0
2. Serious complication of vomiting
3. Emetic
4. Prevents a sharp change in the pH of fluids
5. Released as a waste product from working muscles (2 words)

CHECK YOUR KNOWLEDGE

Multiple Choice

Select the best answer.

1. A pH lower than 7.0 indicates:
   a. An acid solution
   b. An alkaline solution
   c. A lower concentration of hydrogen than hydroxide ions
   d. Both A and C

2. The overall pH range is expressed numerically on what is called a(n):
   a. pH calculator
   b. Acid-base numerator
   c. Logarithmic scale of 1-14
   d. Hydrogen-hydroxide value indicator

3. Chemical substances that prevent a sharp change in the pH of a fluid when an acid or base is added to it are called:
   a. Buffers
   b. Ketone bodies
   c. Enzymes
   d. Fixed acids

4. Lactic acid and other "fixed" acids are buffered by _____ in the blood.
   a. Hydrochloric acid
   b. Carbonic acid
   c. Carbon dioxide
   d. Sodium bicarbonate

5. Which of the following occurs during the vomit reflex?
   a. Hypersalivation
   b. Glottis opens
   c. Diaphragm relaxes
   d. Cardiac sphincter contracts

6. Which of the following is responsible for regulating the pH of body fluids?
   a. Respiratory mechanism
   b. Urinary mechanism
   c. Buffer mechanism
   d. All of the above

7. Which of the following statements regarding metabolic disturbances is correct?
   a. Metabolic acidosis is a bicarbonate deficit.
   b. Metabolic alkalosis is a bicarbonate excess.
   c. Metabolic alkalosis is a complication of severe vomiting.
   d. All of the above are correct.

8. Which of the following statements regarding respiratory disturbances is correct?
   a. Depression of the respiratory center by drugs or disease can cause respiratory acidosis.
   b. Hyperventilation can result in respiratory alkalosis.
   c. Excess carbon dioxide in the arterial blood contributes to respiratory acidosis.
   d. All of the above are correct.

9. The key to acid-base balance is the:
   a. CO_2 ratio
   b. Buffer mechanism
   c. Ratio of respirations to blood pH levels
   d. Ratio of $NaHCO_3$ to H_2CO_3

10. Which statement is false regarding the blood after expired respirations?
    a. It has fewer hydrogen ions than deoxygenated blood entering pulmonary circulation.
    b. It has a higher pH than does the deoxygenated blood entering the pulmonary circulation.
    c. It contains less H_2CO_3 than does the deoxygenated blood entering pulmonary circulation.
    d. The lungs remove approximately 10 L of carbonic acid each day from the venous blood by the elimination of CO_2.

Matching

Select the most correct answer from column B for each statement in column A. (Only one answer is correct.)

Column A

11. _____ Blood

12. _____ Gastric juice

13. _____ Alkalosis

14. _____ "Fixed" acid

15. _____ Buffer

16. _____ Ketone bodies

17. _____ Carbonic anhydrase

18. _____ Acidosis

19. _____ Hyperventilation

20. _____ Emphysema

Column B

a. Excessive fat metabolism

b. Red blood cell enzyme

c. Acid

d. pH imbalance

e. Lactic acid

f. Baking soda

g. Alkaline

h. Respiratory acidosis

i. Arterial blood pH greater than 7.45

j. Respiratory alkalosis

CHAPTER 21
Reproductive System

The reproductive system consists of those organs that participate in perpetuating the species. It is a unique body system in that its organs differ between the two sexes and yet they work toward the same goal: creating a new life. Of interest also is the fact that this system is the only one not necessary to the survival of the individual, and yet survival of the species depends on its proper functioning. The male reproductive system is divided into the external genitals, the testes, the duct system, and accessory glands. The testes, or gonads, are considered essential organs because they produce the sex cells, sperm, that join with the female sex cells, ova, to form a new human being. They also secrete the male sex hormone, testosterone, which is responsible for the physical transformation of a boy to a man.

Sperm are formed in the testes by the seminiferous tubules. From there they enter a long narrow duct, the epididymis. They continue onward through the vas deferens into the ejaculatory duct, down the urethra, and out of the body. Throughout this journey, various glands secrete substances that add motility to the sperm and create a chemical environment conducive to reproduction.

The female reproductive system is truly extraordinary and diverse. It produces ova, receives the penis and sperm during intercourse, serves as the site of conception, houses and feeds the embryo during prenatal development, and nourishes the infant after birth.

Because of its diversity, the physiology of the female is generally considered to be more complex than that of the male. Much of the activity of this system revolves around the menstrual cycle and the monthly preparation that the female undergoes for a possible pregnancy.

The organs of the female system are divided into essential organs and accessory organs of reproduction. The essential organs of the female are the ovaries. Just as with the male, the essential organs of the female are referred to as the *gonads*. The gonads of both sexes produce the sex cells. In the male, the gonads produce the sperm and in the female they produce the ova. The gonads are also responsible for producing the hormones in each sex necessary for the appearance of the secondary sex characteristics.

The menstrual cycle of the female typically covers a period of 28 days. Each cycle consists of three phases: the menstrual period, the postmenstrual phase, and the premenstrual phase. Changes in the blood levels of the hormones that are responsible for the menstrual cycle also cause physical and emotional changes in the female. Knowledge of these phenomena and this system, in both the male and the female, are necessary to complete your understanding of the reproductive system.

TOPICS FOR REVIEW

Before progressing to Chapter 22, you should familiarize yourself with the structure and function of the organs of the male and female reproductive systems. Your review should include emphasis on the gross and microscopic structure of the testes and the production of sperm and testosterone. Your study should continue by tracing and understanding the pathway of a sperm cell from formation to expulsion from the body.

You should then familiarize yourself with the structure and function of the organs of the female reproductive system. Your review should include emphasis on the development of a mature ovum from ovarian follicles and should additionally concentrate on the phases and occurrences in a typical 28-day menstrual cycle.

SEXUAL REPRODUCTION—MALE REPRODUCTIVE SYSTEM—STRUCTURAL PLAN

Match the term on the left with the proper selection on the right.

Group A

1. _____ Testes
2. _____ Spermatozoa
3. _____ Ova
4. _____ Penis
5. _____ Zygote

a. Fertilized ovum
b. Accessory organ
c. Male sex cell
d. Gonads
e. Gamete

Group B

6. _____ Testes
7. _____ Bulbourethral
8. _____ Asexual
9. _____ External genitalia
10. _____ Prostate

a. Cowper gland
b. Scrotum
c. Essential organ
d. Single parent
e. Accessory organ

➡ *If you had difficulty with this section, review pages 459-460.*

TESTES

Multiple Choice

Select the best answer.

11. The testes are surrounded by a tough membrane called the:
    a. Vas deferens
    b. Tunica albuginea
    c. Septum
    d. Seminiferous membrane

12. The _____ lie near the septa that separate the lobules.
    a. Vas deferens
    b. Sperm
    c. Interstitial cells
    d. Nerves

13. Sperm are found in the walls of the:
    a. Seminiferous tubule
    b. Interstitial cells
    c. Septum
    d. Blood vessels

14. An undescended testicle is called a(n):
    a. Orchidalgia
    b. Orchidorrhaphy
    c. Orchichorea
    d. Cryptorchidism

15. The structure(s) that produce(s) testosterone is (are) the:
    a. Seminiferous tubules
    b. Prostate gland
    c. Bulbourethral glands
    d. Pituitary gland
    e. Interstitial cells

16. The part of the sperm that contains genetic information that will be inherited is the:
    a. Tail
    b. Neck
    c. Middle piece
    d. Head
    e. Acrosome

17. Which one of the following is *not* a function of testosterone?
    a. It causes a deepening of the voice.
    b. It promotes the development of the male accessory organs.
    c. It has a stimulatory effect on protein catabolism.
    d. It causes greater muscular development and strength.

18. Sperm production is called:
    a. Spermatogonia
    b. Spermatids
    c. Spermatogenesis
    d. Spermatocyte

19. The section of the sperm that contains enzymes that enable it to break down the covering of the ovum and permit entry should contact occur is the:
    a. Acrosome
    b. Midpiece
    c. Tail
    d. Stem

20. Descent of the testes usually occurs about:
    a. Two months after birth
    b. Two months before birth
    c. Two months after conception
    d. Two years after birth
    e. None of the above

Fill in the blanks.

The (21) _____ are the gonads of the male. From puberty on, the seminiferous tubules are continuously forming (22) _____. Any of these cells may join with the female sex cell, the (23) _____, to become a zygote.

Another function of the testes is to secrete the male hormone (24) _____, which transforms a boy to a man. This hormone is secreted by the (25) _____ _____ of the testes. A good way to remember testosterone's functions is to think of it as "the (26) _____ hormone" and "the (27) _____ hormone."

 If you had difficulty with this section, review pages 460-464.

REPRODUCTIVE DUCTS—ACCESSORY—GLANDS—EXTERNAL—GENITALS

Choose the correct term and write the letter in the space next to the appropriate definition below.

a. Epididymis   f. Prostate gland
b. Vas deferens   g. Cowper gland
c. Ejaculatory duct   h. Prostatectomy
d. Prepuce   i. Semen
e. Seminal vesicles   j. Scrotum

28. _____ Continuation of ducts that start in epididymis

29. _____ Procedure performed for benign prostatic hypertrophy

30. _____ Also known as *bulbourethral*

31. _____ Coiled tube that lies along the top and behind the testes

32. _____ Doughnut-shaped gland beneath bladder

33. _____ Continuation of vas deferens

34. _____ Mixture of sperm and secretions of accessory sex glands

35. _____ Contributes 60% of the seminal fluid volume

36. _____ Removed during circumcision

37. _____ External genitalia

➡ *If you had difficulty with this section, review pages 464-466.*

FEMALE REPRODUCTIVE SYSTEM—STRUCTURAL PLAN

Match the term on the left with the proper selection on the right.

38. _____ Ovaries   a. External genitals
                         b. Accessory sex glands
39. _____ Vagina   c. Accessory duct
40. _____ Vestibular   d. Gonads
41. _____ Vulva   e. Sex cells
42. _____ Ova

Select the correct term from the options given and write the letter in the answer blank.

a. External structure
b. Internal structure

43. _____ Mons pubis

44. _____ Vagina

45. _____ Labia majora

46. _____ Uterine tubes

47. _____ Vestibule

48. _____ Clitoris

49. _____ Labia minora

50. _____ Ovaries

➡ *If you had difficulty with this section, review pages 466-473.*

OVARIES

Fill in the blanks.

The ovaries are the (51) _____ of the female. They have two main functions. The first is the production of the female sex cell. This process is called (52) _____. The specialized type of cell division that occurs during sexual cell reproduction is known as (53) _____. The ovum is the body's largest cell and has (54) _____ _____ the number of chromosomes found in other body cells. At the time of (55) _____, the sex cells from both parents fuse and (56) _____ chromosomes are united.

The second major function of the ovaries is to secrete the sex hormones (57) _____ and (58) _____. Estrogen is the sex hormone that causes the development and maintenance of the female (59) _____ _____ _____. Progesterone acts with estrogen to help initiate the (60) _____ _____ in girls entering (61) _____.

➡ *If you had difficulty with this section, review pages 467-468.*

FEMALE REPRODUCTIVE DUCTS

Select the correct term from the options given and write the letter in the answer blank.

a. Uterine tubes
b. Uterus
c. Vagina

62. _____ Ectopic pregnancy

63. _____ Lining known as *endometrium*

64. _____ Terminal end of birth canal

65. _____ Site of menstruation

66. _____ Approximately 4 inches in length

67. _____ Consists of body, fundus, and cervix

68. _____ Site of fertilization

69. _____ Also known as *oviduct*

70. _____ Entranceway for sperm

71. _____ Total hysterectomy

➡ *If you had difficulty with this section, review pages 466-471.*

ACCESSORY GLANDS—EXTERNAL GENITALS OF THE FEMALE

Match the term on the left with the proper selection on the right.

Group A

72. _____ Bartholin glands

73. _____ Breasts

74. _____ Alveoli

75. _____ Lactiferous ducts

76. _____ Areola

a. Colored area around nipple
b. Grapelike clusters of milk-secreting cells
c. Drain alveoli
d. Secretes lubricating fluid
e. Primarily fat tissue

Group B

77. _____ Mons pubis

78. _____ Labia majora

79. _____ Clitoris

80. _____ Vestibule

81. _____ Episiotomy

a. "Large lips"
b. Area between labia minora
c. Surgical procedure
d. Composed of erectile tissue
e. Pad of fat over the symphysis pubis

➜ *If you had difficulty with this section, review pages 471-473.*

MENSTRUAL CYCLE

True or False

If the statement is true, insert "T" in the answer blank. If the statement is false, correct the statement by circling the incorrect term and writing the correct term in the answer blank.

82. _____ "Climacteric" is the scientific name for the beginning of the menses.

83. _____ As a general rule, several ovum mature each month during the 30-40 years that a woman has menstrual periods.

84. _____ Ovulation occurs 28 days before the next menstrual period begins.

85. _____ The first day of ovulation is considered the first day of the cycle.

86. _____ A woman's fertile period lasts only a few days of each month.

87. _____ The control of the menstrual cycle lies in the posterior pituitary gland.

Matching

Write the letter of the correct hormone in the blank next to the appropriate description.

a. FSH
b. LH

88. _____ Ovulating hormone

89. _____ Secreted during first days of menstrual cycle

90. _____ Secreted after estrogen level of blood increases

91. _____ Causes final maturation of follicle and ovum

92. _____ Birth control pills suppress this hormone

➜ *If you had difficulty with this section, review pages 473-477.*

UNSCRAMBLE THE WORDS

Unscramble the circled letters and fill in the statement.

93. **U L A V V**

94. **T S T S E E**

95. **M N S S E E**

96. **A I E I F M B R**

97. **C U E R P P E**

Where Kathleen displayed the flowers from her husband.

98.

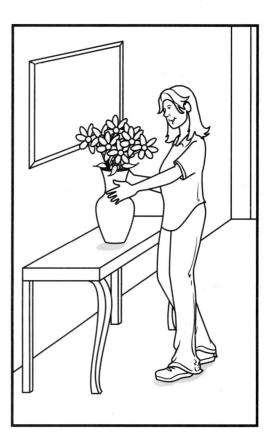

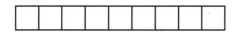

APPLYING WHAT YOU KNOW

99. Mr. Belinki is going to the hospital for the surgical removal of his testes. As a result of this surgery, will Mr. Belinki be impotent?

100. When baby Ross was born, the pediatrician discovered that his left testicle had not descended into the scrotum. If this situation is not corrected soon, might baby Ross be sterile or impotent?

101. Ms. Satin contracted gonorrhea. By the time she made an appointment to see her doctor, it had spread to her abdominal organs. How is this possible when gonorrhea is a disease of the reproductive system?

102. Mrs. Harlan was having a bilateral oophorectomy. Is this a sterilization procedure? Will she experience menopause?

103. Christie had a total hysterectomy. Will she experience menopause?

104. WORD FIND

Can you find 18 terms from this chapter in the box of letters? Words may be spelled top to bottom, bottom to top, right to left, left to right, or diagonally.

```
M  K  O  V  I  D  U  C  T  S  E  D  H  G
S  E  I  R  A  V  O  I  F  U  T  G  L  L
I  N  H  Z  H  M  P  M  K  O  H  I  C  W
D  D  V  A  S  D  E  F  E  R  E  N  S  H
I  O  A  C  C  I  P  J  V  E  H  Y  D  S
H  M  G  R  R  B  M  N  X  F  G  Y  I  O
C  E  I  O  O  E  Z  Y  T  I  C  S  T  E
R  T  N  S  T  P  S  D  D  N  O  V  A  D
O  R  A  O  U  W  E  B  A  I  J  S  M  Z
T  I  C  M  M  E  Y  N  E  M  D  L  R  V
P  U  A  E  U  D  G  M  I  E  H  I  E  H
Y  M  O  T  C  E  T  A  T  S  O  R  P  B
R  P  E  E  R  M  N  E  G  O  R  T  S  E
C  O  W  P  E  R  S  I  N  X  K  E  A  P
```

Acrosome	Meiosis	Scrotum
Cowpers	Ovaries	Seminiferous
Cryptorchidism	Oviducts	Sperm
Endometrium	Penis	Spermatids
Epididymis	Pregnancy	Vagina
Estrogen	Prostatectomy	Vas deferens

? **DID YOU KNOW?**

- The testes produce approximately 500 million sperm per day. Every 2-3 months they produce enough cells to populate the entire earth.
- There are an estimated 925,000 daily occurrences of sexually transmitted disease transmission and 550,000 daily pregnancies worldwide.
- During menstruation, the sensitivity of a woman's middle finger is reduced.
- The lifespan of a sperm on the average is 36 hours. The lifespan of an ovum on the average is 12-24 hours.

REPRODUCTIVE SYSTEMS

Fill in the crossword puzzle.

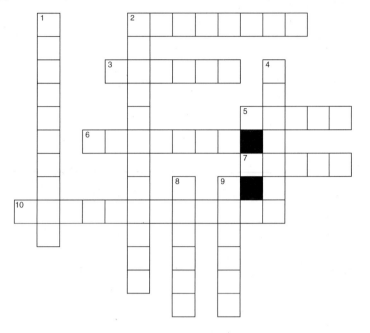

ACROSS
2. Female erectile tissue
3. Colored area around nipple
5. Male reproductive fluid
6. Sex cells
7. Female external genitalia
10. Male sex hormone

DOWN
1. Failure to have a menstrual period
2. Surgical removal of foreskin
4. Foreskin
8. Menstrual period
9. Essential organs of reproduction

CHECK YOUR KNOWLEDGE

Multiple Choice

Select the best answer.

1. Which of the following is *not* an accessory organ of the male reproductive system?
   a. Gonads
   b. Prostate gland
   c. Scrotum
   d. Seminal vesicle

2. The acrosome:
   a. Contains the ATP to provide energy for the sperm
   b. Lies within the nucleus of the sperm
   c. Is responsible for sperm reproduction
   d. Contains enzymes that enable the sperm to enter the ovum

3. Which of the following contribute to the production of seminal fluid?
   a. Seminal vesicles
   b. Prostate gland
   c. Bulbourethral glands
   d. All of the above

4. Sperm mature and develop their ability to move or swim in the:
   a. Ductus deferens
   b. Ejaculatory duct
   c. Epididymis
   d. Cowper glands

5. The bulbourethral glands:
   a. Are shaped like a doughnut
   b. Contribute 60% of the seminal fluid
   c. Secrete "pre-ejaculate"
   d. Pass through the inguinal canal as part of the spermatic cord

6. A mature ovum in its sac is sometimes called a(n):
   a. Graafian follicle
   b. Corpus luteum
   c. Oocyte
   d. Oogenesis

7. Progesterone:
   a. Initiates the first menstrual cycle
   b. Is produced by the corpus luteum
   c. Is responsible for the appearance of pubic hair and breast development
   d. All of the above

8. The external genitalia include all of the following *except:*
   a. Hymen
   b. Clitoris
   c. Lactiferous ducts
   d. Labia minora

9. Testosterone is produced by the:
   a. Interstitial cells
   b. Seminiferous tubules
   c. Process of meiosis
   d. Tunica albuginea

10. Which of the following analogous features of the reproductive systems is correct?
    a. Ovaries to testes
    b. Estrogen and progesterone to testosterone
    c. Clitoris and vulva to penis and scrotum
    d. All of the above

Matching

Select the most correct answer from column B for each statement in column A. (Only one answer is correct.)

Column A

11. _____ Sex cells
12. _____ Sperm stem cells
13. _____ Testosterone
14. _____ Penis
15. _____ Scrotum
16. _____ Ovulating hormone
17. _____ Sperm formation
18. _____ Menses
19. _____ Breasts
20. _____ Vestibule

Column B

a. Spermatogonia
b. FSH
c. Gametes
d. Menarche
e. LH
f. Male external genitalia
g. Prepuce
h. Masculinizes
i. Female external genitalia
j. Areola

MALE REPRODUCTIVE ORGANS

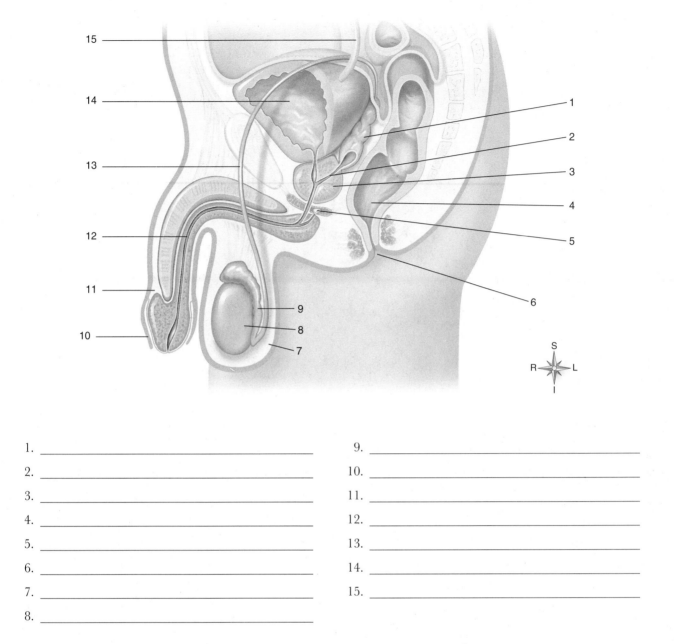

1. _____
2. _____
3. _____
4. _____
5. _____
6. _____
7. _____
8. _____

9. _____
10. _____
11. _____
12. _____
13. _____
14. _____
15. _____

TUBULES OF TESTIS AND EPIDIDYMIS

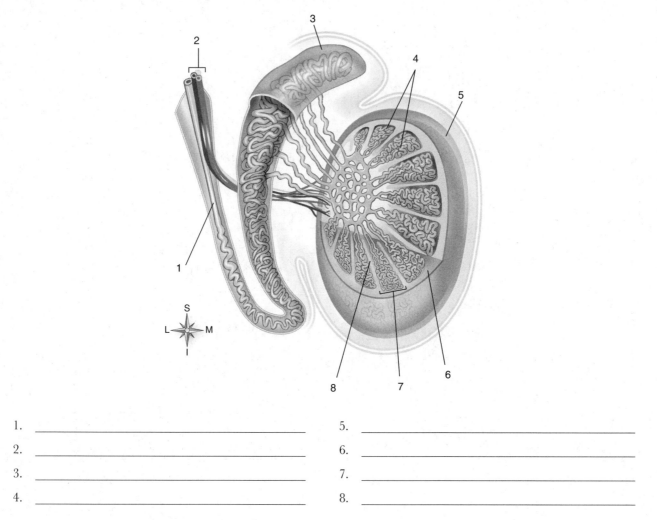

1. _____   5. _____
2. _____   6. _____
3. _____   7. _____
4. _____   8. _____

VULVA

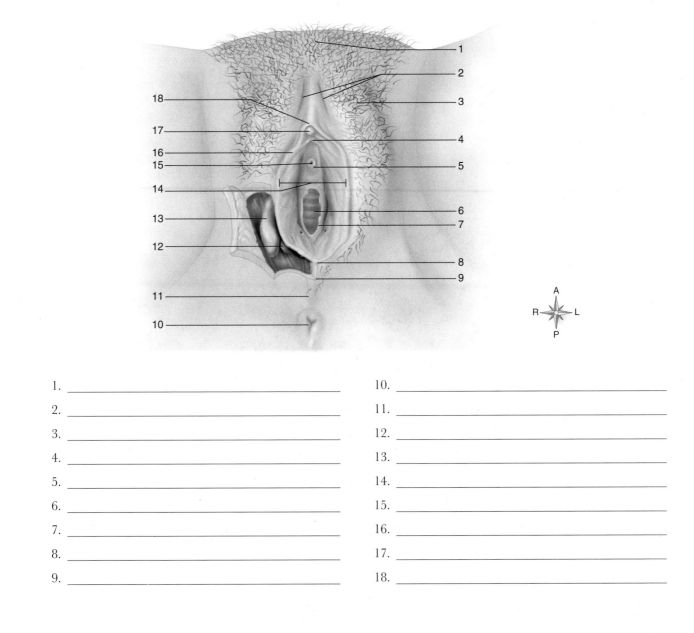

1. _____

2. _____

3. _____

4. _____

5. _____

6. _____

7. _____

8. _____

9. _____

10. _____

11. _____

12. _____

13. _____

14. _____

15. _____

16. _____

17. _____

18. _____

BREAST

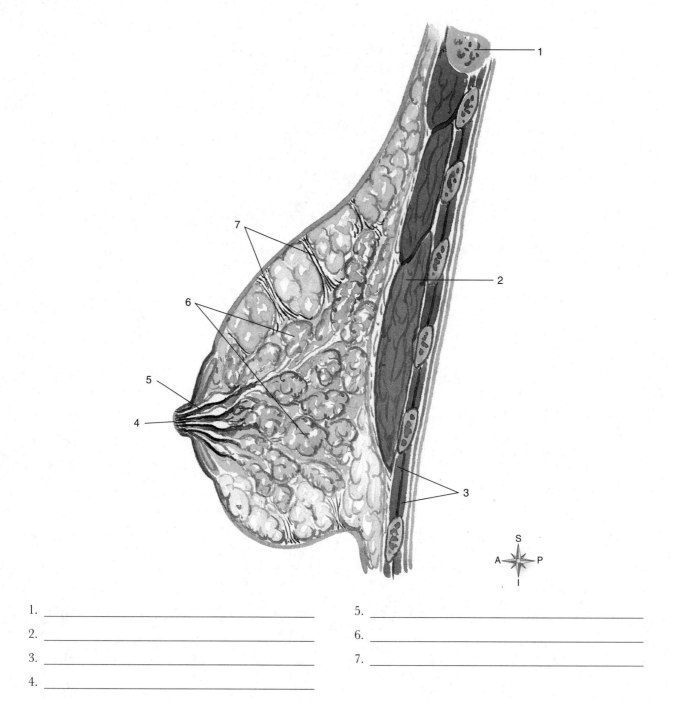

1. _____

2. _____

3. _____

4. _____

5. _____

6. _____

7. _____

FEMALE PELVIS

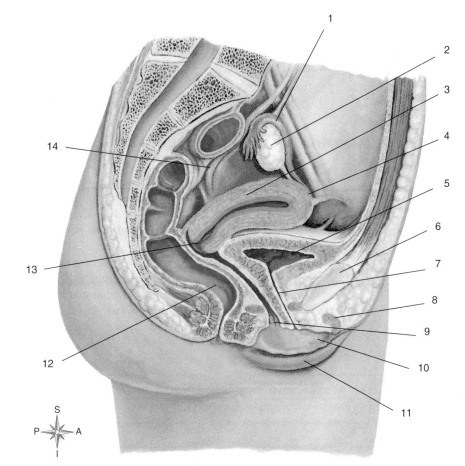

1. _____
2. _____
3. _____
4. _____
5. _____
6. _____
7. _____

8. _____
9. _____
10. _____
11. _____
12. _____
13. _____
14. _____

Matching

Choose the correct term and write the letter in the space next to the appropriate definition below.

a. Laparoscope   f. Endoderm
b. Gestation   g. In vitro
c. Antenatal   h. Parturition
d. Histogenesis   i. Embryonic phase
e. Quickening   j. Ultrasonogram

11. _____ "Within a glass"

12. _____ Inside germ layer

13. _____ Before birth

14. _____ Length of pregnancy

15. _____ Fiberoptic viewing instrument

16. _____ Process of birth

17. _____ First fetal movement

18. _____ Study of how the primary germ layers develop into many different kinds of tissues

19. _____ Fertilization until the end of the eighth week of gestation

20. _____ Monitors the progress of the developing fetus

➡ *If you had difficulty with this section, review pages 484-494.*

POSTNATAL PERIOD

Multiple Choice

Select the best answer.

21. During the postnatal period:
    a. The head becomes proportionately smaller
    b. Thoracic and abdominal contours change from round to elliptical
    c. The legs become proportionately longer
    d. The trunk becomes proportionately shorter
    e. All of the above

22. The period of infancy starts at birth and lasts about:
    a. 4 weeks
    b. 4 months
    c. 10 weeks
    d. 12 months
    e. 18 months

23. The lumbar curvature of the spine appears _____ months after birth.
    a. 1-10
    b. 5-8
    c. 8-12
    d. 11-15
    e. 12-18

24. During the first 4 months, the birth weight will:
    a. Double
    b. Triple
    c. Quadruple
    d. None of the above

25. At the end of the first year, the weight of the baby will have:
    a. Doubled
    b. Tripled
    c. Quadrupled
    d. None of the above

26. The infant is capable of following a moving object with its eyes at:
    a. 2 days
    b. 2 weeks
    c. 2 months
    d. 4 months
    e. 10 months

27. The infant can lift its head and raise its chest at:
    a. 2 months
    b. 3 months
    c. 4 months
    d. 10 months

28. The infant can crawl at the age of:
    a. 2 months
    b. 3 months
    c. 4 months
    d. 10 months
    e. 12 months

29. The infant can stand alone at the age of:
    a. 2 months
    b. 3 months
    c. 4 months
    d. 10 months
    e. 12 months

30. The permanent teeth, with the exception of the third molar, have all erupted by age _____ years.
    a. 6
    b. 8
    c. 12
    d. 14
    e. None of the above

31. Puberty starts at age _____ years in boys.
    a. 10-13
    b. 12-14
    c. 14-16
    d. None of the above

32. Most girls begin breast development at about age:
    a. 8
    b. 9
    c. 10
    d. 11
    e. 12

33. The growth spurt is generally complete by age _____ in males.
    a. 14
    b. 15
    c. 16
    d. 18

34. An average age at which girls begin to menstruate is _____ years.
    a. 10-12
    b. 11-12
    c. 12-13
    d. 13-14
    e. 14-15

35. The first sign of puberty in boys is:
    a. Facial hair
    b. Increased muscle mass
    c. Pubic hair
    d. Deepening of the voice
    e. Increased testicular enlargement

Matching

Write the letter of the correct word in the blank next to the appropriate definition.

a. Neonatology   f. Postnatal
b. Neonatal   g. Infancy
c. Adolescence   h. Childhood
d. Deciduous   i. Senescence
e. Puberty

36. _____ Begins at birth and lasts until death

37. _____ Concerned with the diagnosis and treatment of disorders of the newborn

38. _____ Teenage years

39. _____ From the end of infancy to puberty

40. _____ Baby teeth

41. _____ First 4 weeks of infancy

42. _____ Secondary sexual characteristics occur

43. _____ Begins at birth and lasts about 18 months

44. _____ Older adulthood

➡ *If you had difficulty with this section, review pages 493-496.*

EFFECTS OF AGING

Fill in the blanks.

45. Old bones develop indistinct and shaggy margins with spurs, a process called _____.

46. A degenerative joint disease common in the older adults is _____.

47. The number of _____ units in the kidney decreases by almost 50% between the ages of 30 and 75.

48. In older adulthood, respiratory efficiency decreases, and a condition known as _____ _____ results.

49. Fatty deposits accumulate in blood vessels as we age, and the result is _____, which narrows the passageway for the flow of blood.

50. Hardening of the arteries, or _____, occurs during the aging process.

51. Another term for high blood pressure is _____.

52. Hardening of the lens is _____.

53. If the lens becomes cloudy and impairs vision, it is called a(n) _____.

54. _____ causes an increase in the pressure within the eyeball and may result in blindness.

➔ *If you had difficulty with this section, review pages 496-499.*

UNSCRAMBLE THE WORDS

Unscramble the circled letters and fill in the statement.

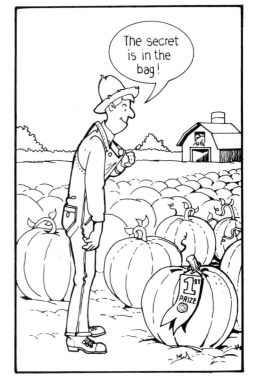

The secret is in the bag!

55. **A N N F C Y I**

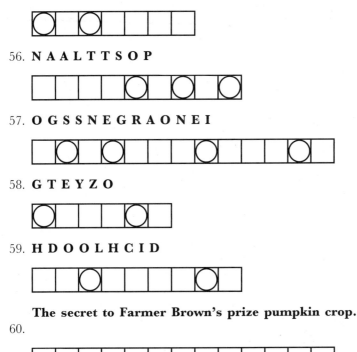

56. **N A A L T T S O P**

57. **O G S S N E G R A O N E I**

58. **G T E Y Z O**

59. **H D O O L H C I D**

The secret to Farmer Brown's prize pumpkin crop.

60.

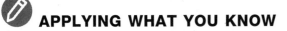

APPLYING WHAT YOU KNOW

61. Heather's mother told the pediatrician during her 1-year visit that Heather had tripled her birth weight, was crawling actively, and could stand alone. Is Heather's development normal, retarded, or advanced?

62. Sharon is 70 years old. She has always enjoyed food and has had a hearty appetite. Lately, however, she has complained that food "just doesn't taste as good anymore." What might be a possible explanation?

63. Mr. Hines, age 78, has noticed hearing problems, but only under certain circumstances. He has difficulty with certain tones, especially high or low tones but has no problem with everyday conversation. What might be a possible explanation?

64. WORD FIND

Can you find 14 terms from the chapter in the box of letters? Words may be spelled top to bottom, bottom to top, right to left, left to right, or diagonally.

```
F  T  P  N  O  I  T  A  T  S  E  G  K  F  U
Z  E  P  O  C  S  O  R  A  P  A  L  H  E  A
E  O  R  I  L  T  O  H  H  O  C  J  V  J  T
C  M  V  T  N  T  I  M  L  N  L  Z  P  U  O
M  A  B  I  I  F  R  M  R  E  D  O  T  C  E
H  Q  C  R  D  L  A  M  E  S  O  D  E  R  M
N  N  M  U  Y  U  I  N  M  F  O  W  G  O  P
K  N  V  T  C  O  Z  C  H  H  F  R  C  N
H  G  Y  R  K  L  T  A  Y  D  U  C  V  P
L  A  T  A  N  T  S  O  P  T  L  U  N  Q  G
Q  N  K  P  Y  Y  S  W  G  A  I  K  E  M  T
U  G  P  Q  N  H  O  Y  X  Y  H  O  Z  B  N
I  Y  T  R  E  B  U  P  L  A  C  E  N  T  A
```

Childhood	Infancy	Parturition
Ectoderm	Laparoscope	Placenta
Embryology	Mesoderm	Postnatal
Fertilization	Morula	Puberty
Gestation	Oviduct	

❓ DID YOU KNOW?

- Brain cells do not regenerate. One beer permanently destroys 10,000 cells.
- A 3-week-old embryo is no larger than a sesame seed. A 1-month-old embryo's body is no heavier than an envelope and a sheet of paper. Its hand is no bigger than a teardrop.
- During pregnancy, the uterus expands to 500 times its normal size.
- From birth to adolescence, selected bones in the human body fuse together. The last bone to fuse is the collarbone, and this occurs between the ages of 18 and 25.

GROWTH, DEVELOPMENT, AND AGING

Fill in the crossword puzzle.

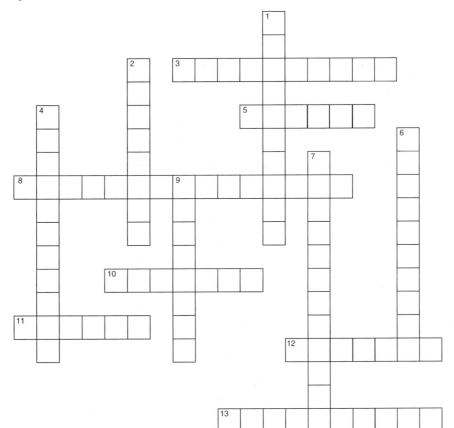

Across
3. Hardening of the lens
5. Fertilized ovum
8. Fatty deposit buildup in walls of arteries
10. Will develop into a fetal membrane in the placenta
11. Name of zygote after 3 days
12. First 4 weeks of infancy
13. Old age

Down
1. Science of the development of the individual before birth
2. Eye disease marked by increased pressure in the eyeball
4. Process of birth
6. Name of zygote after implantation
7. Process of how germ layers develop into tissues
9. Cloudy lens

CHECK YOUR KNOWLEDGE

Multiple Choice

Select the best answer.

1. The prenatal period begins:
   a. After implantation
   b. 4 weeks after gestation
   c. At conception
   d. 10 days after conception

2. By the time the developing embryo reaches the uterus, it is a:
   a. Morula
   b. Zygote
   c. Fetus
   d. Blastocyst

3. The chorion develops into the:
   a. Morula
   b. Zygote
   c. Fetus
   d. Placenta

4. Fertilization most often occurs in the:
   a. Outer one-third of the oviduct
   b. Inner one-third of the oviduct
   c. Uterus
   d. Vagina

5. The embryonic phase of development extends from fertilization until the end of week _____ of gestation.
   a. 2
   b. 4
   c. 6
   d. 8

6. The primary germ layers include the:
   a. Endoderm
   b. Ectoderm
   c. Mesoderm
   d. All of the above

7. The stage of labor that begins from the onset of uterine contractions until dilation of the cervix is complete is called:
   a. Parturition
   b. Transition
   c. Stage one
   d. Stage two

8. All organ systems are complete and in place by:
   a. 4 months of gestation
   b. 35 days of gestation
   c. 7 months of gestation
   d. 8 months of gestation

9. The initial stimulus to breathe when an infant is born results from the:
   a. Doctor shocking the baby by slapping the buttocks
   b. Cold new environment shocking the respiratory system
   c. Increasing amounts of carbon dioxide that accumulate in the blood after the umbilical cord is cut following delivery
   d. Baby's sudden change of position after delivery

10. Adulthood is characterized by:
    a. A period of rapid growth
    b. Maintenance of existing body tissues
    c. Senescence
    d. None of the above

Matching

Select the most correct answer from column B for each statement in column A. (Only one answer is correct.)

Column A

11. _____ Embryology
12. _____ Zygote
13. _____ Gestation period
14. _____ Older adult
15. _____ Teratogens
16. _____ Quickening
17. _____ Lipping
18. _____ Presbyopia
19. _____ Gerontology
20. _____ Infancy

Column B

a. Study of aging
b. First 18 months of life
c. Trimesters
d. Fetal movement
e. Prenatal science
f. "Old eye"
g. Fertilized ovum
h. Factors that cause birth defects
i. Senescence
j. Bone spurs

FERTILIZATION AND IMPLANTATION

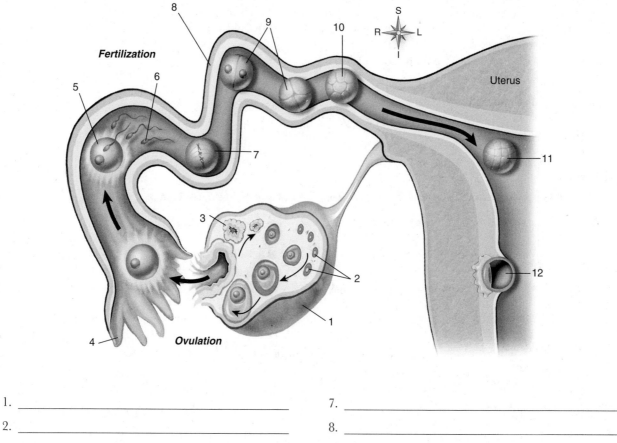

1. _____

2. _____

3. _____

4. _____

5. _____

6. _____

7. _____

8. _____

9. _____

10. _____

11. _____

12. _____

Answer Key

CHAPTER 1
INTRODUCTION TO THE BODY

Fill in the Blanks

1. Scientific method, p. 4
2. Hypothesis, p. 4
3. Experimentation, p. 4
4. Test group, p. 4
5. Control group, p. 4

True or False

6. T
7. Meter, not centimeter
8. T
9. T
10. Micron, not centron

Matching

11. d, p. 5
12. e, p. 6
13. a, p. 6
14. c, p. 6
15. b, p. 6

Matching

16. c, p. 7
17. a, p. 7
18. e, p. 7
19. d, p. 7
20. b, p. 7

Crossword

21. Inferior
22. Transverse
23. Medial
24. Superior
25. Ventral
26. Lateral
27. Distal

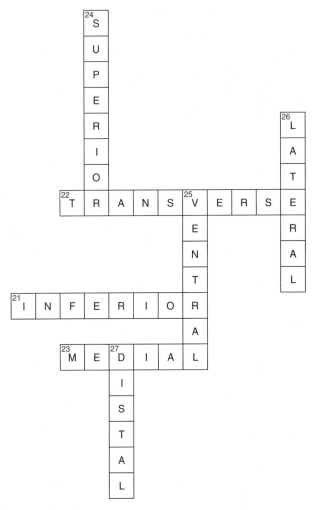

Did you notice that the answers were arranged as they appear on the human body?

Circle the Correct Answer

28. Inferior, p. 7
29. Anterior, p. 7
30. Lateral, p. 7
31. Proximal, p. 7
32. Superficial, p. 7
33. Equal, p. 9
34. Anterior and posterior, p. 9
35. Upper and lower, p. 9
36. Frontal, p. 9

Select the Correct Term

37. a, p. 9
38. b, p. 9
39. a, p. 9
40. a, p. 9
41. a, p. 9
42. b, p. 9
43. a, p. 9

Circle the One That Does Not Belong

44. Extremities (the others refer to the axial portions)
45. Cephalic (the others refer to the arm)
46. Plantar (the others refer to the face)
47. Carpal (the others refer to the leg or foot)
48. Tarsal (the others refer to the skull)

Fill in the Blanks

49. Survival, p. 13
50. Internal environment, p. 13
51. Feedback loop, p. 14
52. Negative, positive, p. 15
53. Stabilize, p. 15
54. Stimulatory, p. 15
55. Developmental processes, p. 16
56. Aging processes, p. 16

Unscramble the Words

57. Axial
58. Physiology
59. Frontal
60. Dorsal
61. Organ

Applying What You Know

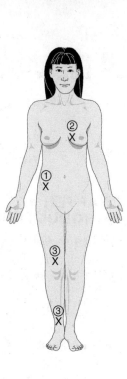

62. #1 on diagram
63. #2 on diagram
64. #3 on diagram
65. In severe bleeding, blood pressure decreases. The heart beats faster to increase the blood pressure back to normal. This increase in heart rate, however, increases the loss of blood, which causes a further drop in blood pressure and an even faster heart rate in an ever-increasing cycle. The increase of blood loss is caused by a positive feedback loop. When this occurs, the immediate emergency care to stop the positive feedback loop would be to apply pressure to the area to stop or slow the loss of blood.
66. WORD FIND

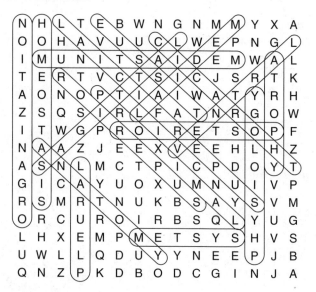

Check Your Knowledge

Multiple Choice

1. a, p. 13
2. d, p. 9
3. b, p. 10
4. d, p. 8
5. a, p. 3
6. c, p. 9
7. c, p. 6
8. a, p. 9
9. c, p. 10
10. b, p. 10
11. d, p. 9
12. b, p. 10
13. c, p. 6
14. a, p. 9
15. d, p. 7
16. c, p. 7

17. d, p. 13
18. d, p. 9
19. a, p. 11
20. c, p. 7

Matching

21. f, p. 9
22. b, p. 13
23. j, p. 9
24. g, p. 3
25. h, p. 7
26. c, p. 9
27. d, p. 11
28. i, p. 7
29. a, p. 9
30. e, p. 6

Dorsal and Ventral Body Cavities

1. Cranial cavity
2. Spinal cavity
3. Thoracic cavity
4. Pleural cavity
5. Mediastinum
6. Diaphragm
7. Abdominal cavity
8. Abdominopelvic cavity
9. Pelvic cavity

Directions and Planes of the Body

1. Superior
2. Proximal
3. Posterior (dorsal)
4. Anterior (ventral)
5. Inferior
6. Sagittal plane
7. Frontal plane
8. Lateral

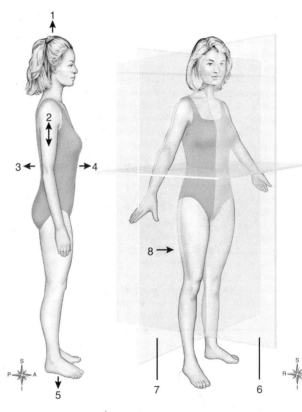

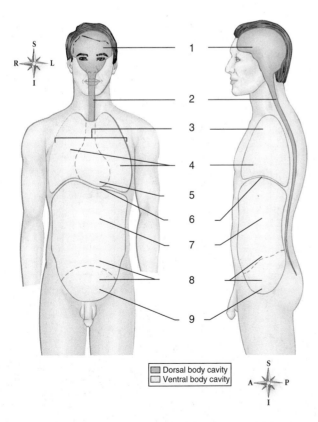

Regions of the Abdomen

1. Right hypochondriac region
2. Epigastric region
3. Left hypochondriac region
4. Right lumbar region
5. Umbilical region
6. Left lumbar region
7. Right iliac (inguinal) region
8. Hypogastric region
9. Left iliac (inguinal) region

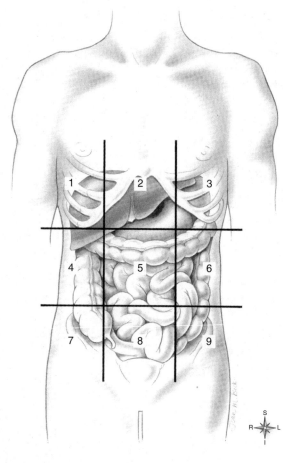

CHAPTER 2
CHEMISTRY OF LIFE

Multiple Choice

1. d, p. 23
2. c, p. 23
3. b, p. 23
4. c, p. 23
5. a, p. 23
6. d, p. 24
7. c, p. 24
8. a, p. 24

True or False

9. T
10. Molecules, not electrons, p. 23
11. T
12. T
13. T

Multiple Choice

14. c, p. 25
15. b, p. 25
16. a, p. 25
17. b, p. 26
18. a, p. 26
19. c, p. 25

Matching

20. h, p. 27
21. b, p. 27
22. e, p. 27
23. a, p. 27
24. g, p. 27
25. l, p. 27
26. j, p. 27
27. c, p. 28
28. d, p. 28
29. f, p. 28
30. k, p. 28
31. i, p. 28

Select the Best Answer

32. a, p. 30
33. b, p. 30
34. d, p. 32
35. b, p. 31
36. c, p. 31
37. a, p. 30
38. a, p. 30
39. b, p. 30
40. c, p. 31
41. d, p. 32

Crossword

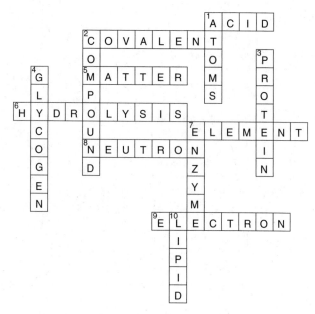

Unscramble the Words

42. Matter
43. Elements
44. Molecules
45. Organic
46. Electrolyte
47. Energy

Applying What You Know

48. Some fats can become solid at room temperature, such as the fat in butter and lard.
49. Radioactive isotopes will be used to measure Carol's thyroid activity. A diagnosis of hyperthyroidism or hypothyroidism will be based on how rapidly or slowly the thyroid absorbs the radioactive iodine and emits radiation.
50. WORD FIND

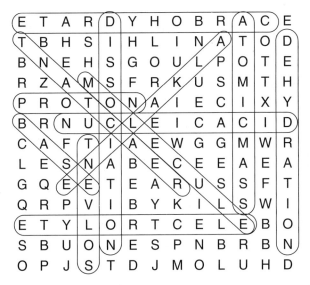

Check Your Knowledge

Fill in the Blanks

1. Biochemistry, p. 23
2. Neutrons, p. 23
3. Higher, p. 24
4. Elements; compounds, p. 24
5. Stable, p. 24
6. Ion, p. 25
7. Inorganic, p. 27
8. Dehydration synthesis, p. 27
9. Chemical equation, p. 28
10. CO_2, p. 28
11. Acids, p. 28
12. Buffers, p. 29
13. Carbohydrate, p. 29
14. Cholesterol, p. 31
15. Structural, p. 32

Multiple Choice

16. a, p. 25
17. a, p. 25
18. b, p. 27
19. d, p. 30
20. c, p. 33

CHAPTER 3 CELLS

Matching

Group A

1. c, p. 43
2. e, p. 42
3. a, p. 42
4. b, p. 42
5. d, p. 46

Group B

6. d, p. 44
7. e, p. 45
8. a, p. 46
9. b, p. 46
10. c, p. 46

Fill in the Blanks

11. Organelles, p. 42
12. Tissue typing, p. 42
13. Cilia, p. 46
14. Cellular respiration, p. 46
15. Ribosomes, p. 44
16. Mitochondria, p. 46
17. Lysosomes, p. 46
18. Golgi apparatus, p. 46
19. Centrioles, p. 46
20. Chromatin granules, p. 47

Multiple Choice

21. a, p. 48
22. d, p. 48
23. b, p. 48
24. d, p. 50
25. c, p. 50
26. a, p. 48
27. b, p. 51
28. c, p. 51
29. d, p. 51
30. a, p. 52
31. b, p. 50
32. a, p. 50

Circle the One That Does Not Belong

33. Uracil (RNA, not DNA, contains the base uracil)
34. Telophase (the others are complementary base pairings of DNA)
35. Anaphase (the others refer to genes and heredity)
36. Thymine (the others refer to RNA)
37. Interphase (the others refer to translation)
38. Prophase (the others refer to anaphase)
39. Prophase (the others refer to interphase)
40. Metaphase (the others refer to telophase)
41. Gene (the others refer to stages of cell division)

Unscramble the Words

42. Interphase
43. Centriole
44. Diffusion
45. Telophase
46. Organelle
47. Translation

Applying What You Know

48.

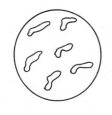

49. Diffusion
50. Absorption of oxygen into Ms. Bence's blood
51. TCCG
52. WORD FIND

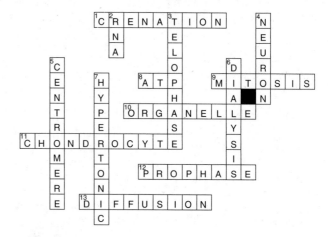

Crossword

Check Your Knowledge

Multiple Choice

1. a, p. 42
2. b, p. 44
3. b, p. 46
4. a, p. 46
5. c, p. 51
6. a, p. 50
7. d, p. 53
8. b, p. 56
9. a, p. 46
10. b, p. 50
11. b, p. 46
12. c, p. 51
13. a, p. 55
14. a, p. 55
15. b, p. 54

Matching

16. f, p. 45
17. g, p. 47
18. j, p. 47
19. c, p. 48
20. a, p. 52
21. b, p. 50
22. i, p. 55
23. h, p. 58
24. d, p. 58
25. e, p. 52

Cell Structure

1. Nucleolus
2. Nuclear envelope
3. Nucleus
4. Microtubules
5. Flagellum
6. Centrioles
7. Centrosome
8. Mitochondrion
9. Golgi apparatus
10. Free ribosomes
11. Plasma membrane
12. Lysosome
13. Microvilli
14. Smooth endoplasmic reticulum
15. Cilia
16. Microfilaments
17. Cytoplasm
18. Ribosome
19. Rough endoplasmic reticulum
20. Chromatin granules
21. Nuclear pore

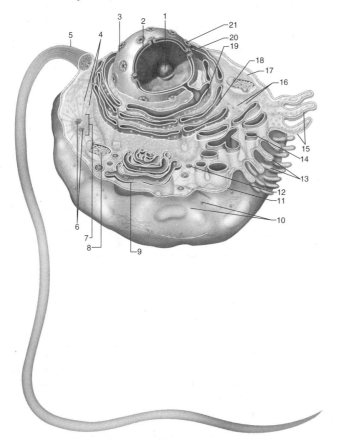

Mitosis

1. Interphase
2. Prophase
3. Metaphase
4. Anaphase
5. Telophase
6. Daughter cells (interphase)

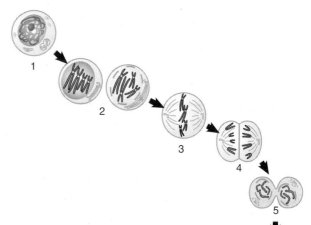

CHAPTER 4
TISSUES

Multiple Choice

1. b, p. 67
2. c, p. 68
3. d, p. 67
4. d, p. 68
5. b, p. 68
6. b, p. 69
7. b, p. 70
8. c, p. 68

Matching

9. b, p. 70
10. e, p. 68
11. a, p. 68
12. c, p. 71
13. d, p. 71
14. f, p. 72

Labeling

1. Simple columnar epithelium (1. Goblet cell, 2. Columnar epithelial cells)
2. Stratified squamous epithelium (1. Superficial squamous epithelial cell, 2. Basal epithelial cell, 3. Basement membrane)
3. Stratified transitional epithelium (1. Basement membrane, 2. Binucleate cell, 3. Stratified transitional epithelial cells)

Multiple Choice

15. a, p. 73
16. d, p. 74
17. a, p. 76
18. c, p. 76
19. a, p. 74
20. d, p. 73

Labeling

4. Adipose tissue (1. Shortage area for fat, 2. Plasma membrane, 3. Nucleus of adipose cell)
5. Dense fibrous connective tissue (1. Nuclei of fiber-producing cells, 2. Bundles of collagenous fibers)
6. Bone tissue (1. Osteon)
7. Blood tissue (1. White blood cell, 2. Matrix [liquid], 3. Red blood cells)

Matching

21. b, p. 77
22. c, p. 78
23. a, p. 77
24. b, p. 77
25. c, p. 78
26. c, p. 78

Labeling

8. Skeletal muscle (1. Striations, 2. Nuclei of muscle fibers, 3. Muscle fiber)
9. Cardiac muscle (1. Nucleus of muscle cell, 2. Intercalated disks)

Matching

27. b, p. 79
28. c, p. 79
29. a, p. 79
30. d, p. 79

Labeling

10. Nervous tissue (1. Nerve cell body, 2. Axon, 3. Dendrites)

31. Fill in the missing areas of the chart.

Tissue	Location	Function
Epithelial		
1.	1a.	1a. Absorption by diffusion of respiratory gases between alveolar air and blood
	1b.	1b. Absorption by diffusion, filtration, and osmosis
2.	2a. Surface of lining of mouth and esophagus	2a.
	2b. Surface of skin	2b.
3.	3. Surface layer of lining of stomach, intestines, and parts of respiratory tract	3.
4. Stratified transitional	4.	4.
5.	5. Surface of lining of trachea	5.
6.	6.	6. Secretion; absorption
Connective		
1.	1. Between other tissues and organs	1.
2. Adipose	2.	2.
3.	3.	3. Flexible but strong connection
4.	4. Skeleton	4.
5.	5. Part of nasal septum, area covering surfaces of bones at joints, larynx wall, rings in trachea, and bronchi, disks between vertebrae and in knee joint, external ear	5.
6.	6.	6. Transportation
7. Hemopoietic tissue	7.	7.
Muscle		
1.	1. Muscles that attach to bones, eyeball muscles, upper third of esophagus	1.
2. Cardiac	2.	
3.	3. Walls of digestive, respiratory, and genitourinary tracts; walls of blood and large lymphatic vessels; ducts of glands; intrinsic eye muscles; arrector muscles of hair	3.
Nervous		
1. Nerve cells	1. Brain and spinal cord, nerves	1.

Unscramble the Words

32. Dendrite
33. Osteon
34. Squamous
35. Stratified
36. Glia
37. Tissues

Applying What You Know

38. Merrily may have exceeded the 18% to 24% desirable body fat composition. Fitness depends more on the percentage and ratio of specific tissue types than the overall amount of tissue present.

39. Holly is too lean. Holly should be in the 20% to 22% range to be considered normal. Holly's obsession may put her at risk for other disease conditions because of the stress to her body of being "too lean."

40. WORD FIND

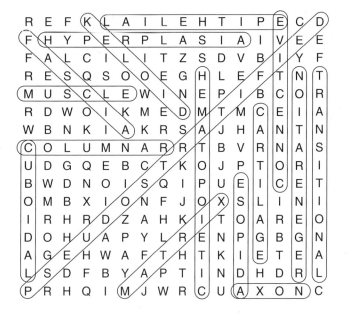

Crossword

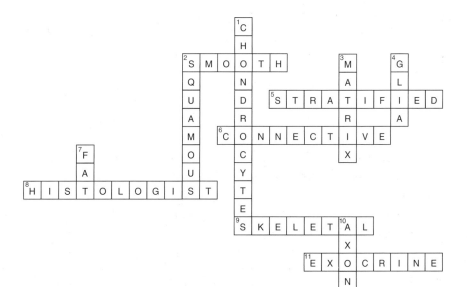

Check Your Knowledge

Labeling

1. Squamous
2. Cuboidal
3. Columnar
4. Simple squamous
5. Simple cuboidal
6. Simple columnar
7. Stratified squamous
8. Pseudostratified columnar

Multiple Choice

9. a, p. 73
10. b, p. 73
11. c, p. 69
12. d, p. 77
13. b, p. 76

Fill in the Blanks

14. Areolar, p. 74
15. Goblet, p. 71
16. Matrix, p. 68
17. Intercalated disks, p. 77
18. Collagen, p. 68
19. Areolar, p. 74
20. Cancellous, p. 76

CHAPTER 5
ORGAN SYSTEMS

Matching

Group A

1. a, p. 86
2. e, p. 87
3. d, p. 87
4. b, p. 88
5. c, p. 88

Group B

6. f, p. 89
7. e, p. 90
8. b, p. 92
9. a, p. 91
10. c, p. 90
11. d, p. 93

Circle the One That Does Not Belong

12. Mouth (the others refer to the respiratory system)
13. Rectum (the others refer to the reproductive system)
14. Pancreas (the others refer to the circulatory system)
15. Pineal (the others refer to the urinary system)
16. Joints (the others refer to the muscular system)
17. Pituitary (the others refer to the nervous system)
18. Tendons (the others refer to the skeletal system)
19. Appendix (the others refer to the endocrine system)
20. Thymus (the others refer to the integumentary system)
21. Trachea (the others refer to the digestive system)
22. Liver (the others refer to the lymphatic system)

Fill in the Missing Areas

System	Organs	Functions
		23. Protection, regulation of body temperature, synthesis of chemicals and hormones, serves as a sense organ
	24. Bones, joints	
		25. Movement, maintains body posture, produces heat
26. Nervous		
	27. Pituitary, thymus, pineal, adrenal, hypothalamus, thyroid, pancreas, parathyroid, ovaries, testes	
		28. Transportation, immunity
	29. Lymph nodes, lymph vessels, thymus, spleen, tonsils	
30. Urinary		
	31. Mouth, pharynx, esophagus, stomach, small and large intestine, rectum, anal canal, teeth, salivary glands, tongue, liver, gallbladder, pancreas, appendix	
32. Respiratory		
	33a. Gonads—testes and ovaries	
	33b. Accessory organs, ducts, and glands (p. 95)	

Unscramble the Words

34. Heart
35. Pineal
36. Nerve
37. Esophagus
38. Nervous

Applying What You Know

39. Endocrinology (endocrine system); gynecology (reproductive system)
40. Sometimes the organs of the endocrine system perform the same general functions as the nervous system, such as communication, integration, and control. The nervous system provides these functions in a rapid, brief, controlled manner by fast traveling nerve impulses. The endocrine system provides the same functions, but in a slower and longer lasting controlled manner by hormone secretion. An example is the secretion of growth hormone that controls the rate of development over long periods of gradual growth.

41. WORD FIND

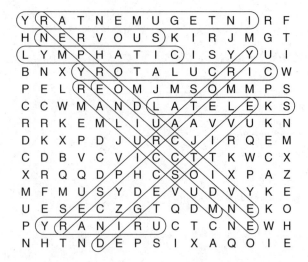

Crossword

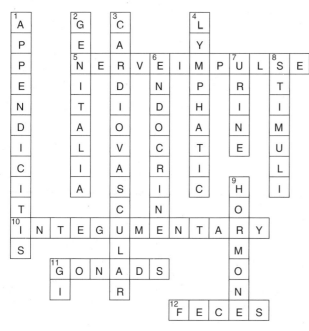

Check Your Knowledge

Multiple Choice

1. d, p. 88
2. c, p. 90
3. c, p. 93
4. b, p. 85
5. d, p. 87
6. a, p. 86
7. b, p. 91
8. a, p. 88
9. a, p. 88
10. c, p. 85

Matching

11. c, p. 86
12. d, p. 89
13. h, p. 90
14. g, p. 93
15. b, p. 92
16. f, p. 91
17. i, p. 93
18. e, p. 90
19. j, p. 88
20. a, p. 88

CHAPTER 6
SKIN AND MEMBRANES

Select the Best Answer

1. b, p. 104
2. d, p. 106
3. c, p. 105
4. a, p. 104
5. b, p. 104
6. d, p. 105
7. c, p. 105
8. c, p. 105

Matching

Group A

9. d, p. 106
10. a, p. 106
11. b, p. 106
12. c, p. 107
13. e, p. 106

Group B

14. a, p. 107
15. d, p. 107
16. e, p. 107
17. c, p. 107
18. b, p. 107

Select the Correct Term

19. a, p. 107
20. b, p. 108
21. b, p. 108
22. a, p. 107
23. a, p. 107
24. b, p. 106
25. b, p. 108
26. b, p. 108
27. b, p. 108
28. a, pp. 107-108 Figure 6-4

Fill in the Blanks

29. Protection, temperature regulation, sense organ activity, excretion and synthesis of vitamin D, p. 110
30. Melanin, p. 107
31. Lanugo, p. 108
32. Hair papillae, p. 109
33. Lunula, p. 109
34. Arrector pili, p. 109
35. Light touch, p. 110
36. Eccrine, p. 110
37. Apocrine, p. 110
38. Sebum, p. 110

Select the Best Answer

39. d, p. 112
40. c, p. 112
41. a, p. 112
42. b, p. 112
43. c, p. 112

Circle the Correct Answer

44. Will not, p. 114
45. Will, p. 114
46. Will not, p. 115
47. 11, p. 114
48. Third, p. 114

Unscramble the Words

49. Epidermis
50. Keratin
51. Hair
52. Lanugo
53. Dehydration
54. Third degree

Applying What You Know

55. 46
56. Pleurisy
57. The skin protects the underlying tissue against invasion by harmful bacteria. With a large percentage of Brian's skin destroyed, he was vulnerable to bacteria, and so he was placed in the cleanest environment possible—isolation. Jenny is required to wear special attire so that the risk of her bringing bacteria to the patient is reduced.
58. WORD FIND

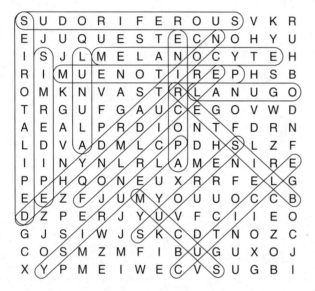

Crossword

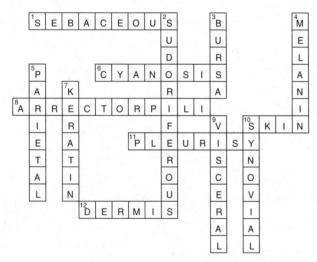

Check Your Knowledge

Multiple Choice

1. a, p. 105
2. b, p. 106
3. a, p. 108
4. d, p. 107
5. b, p. 107
6. d, p. 109
7. b, p. 110
8. b, p. 109
9. c, p. 110
10. b, p. 110

Matching

11. c, p. 104
12. d, p. 104
13. b, p. 104
14. g, p. 105
15. i, p. 105
16. h, p. 107
17. j, p. 108
18. e, p. 109
19. a, p. 110
20. f, p. 110

Completion

21. a, p. 112
22. h, p. 112
23. b, p. 104
24. f, p. 105
25. i, p. 114
26. e, p. 114
27. g, p. 114
28. d, p. 115
29. j, p. 110
30. c, p. 110

Longitudinal Section of the Skin

1. Dermal papilla
2. Stratum corneum
3. Stratum germinativum
4. Openings of sweat ducts
5. Sweat gland
6. Cutaneous nerve
7. Papilla of hair
8. Lamellar (Pacini) corpuscle
9. Hair follicle
10. Arrector muscle
11. Tactile (Meissner's) corpuscle
12. Subcutaneous tissue
13. Dermis
14. Epidermis
15. Sebaceous (oil) gland
16. Hair shaft

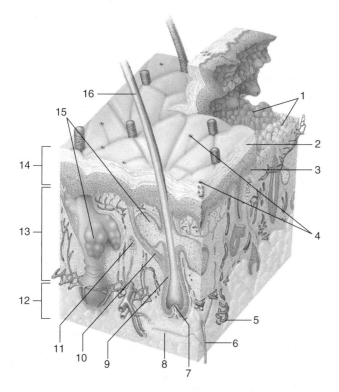

"Rule of Nines" for Estimating Skin Surface Burned

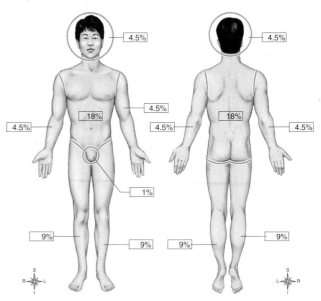

CHAPTER 7 SKELETAL SYSTEM

Fill in the Blanks

1. 4, p. 124
2. Medullary cavity, p. 125
3. Articular cartilage p. 125
4. Endosteum, p. 125
5. Hemopoiesis, p. 124
6. Red bone marrow, p. 124
7. Periosteum, p. 125
8. Elderly white females, p. 129
9. Calcium, p. 124
10. Move, p. 124

Matching

Group A

11. d, p. 125
12. b, p. 125
13. e, p. 125
14. a, p. 125
15. c, p. 125

Group B

16. d, p. 125
17. a, p. 125
18. e, p. 125
19. b, p. 125
20. c, p. 125

True or False

21. T
22. Epiphyses, not diaphyses, p. 127
23. Osteoblasts, not osteoclasts, p. 127
24. T
25. Increase, not decrease, p. 127
26. Juvenile, not adult, p. 127
27. Diaphysis, not articulation, p. 127
28. T
29. Ceases, not begins, p. 127
30. T

Multiple Choice

31. a, p. 136
32. d, p. 131
33. a, p. 135
34. d, p. 135
35. c, p. 138
36. c, p. 140
37. d, p. 138
38. d, p. 140
39. a, p. 140
40. b, p. 131
41. a, p. 135
42. b, p. 138
43. b, p. 135
44. b, p. 136
45. c, p. 138
46. a, p. 139
47. d, p. 131
48. c, p. 133
49. c, p. 131

Circle the One That Does Not Belong

50. Coxal bone (the others refer to the spine)
51. Axial (the others refer to the appendicular skeleton)
52. Maxilla (the others refer to the cranial bones)
53. Ribs (the others refer to the shoulder girdle)
54. Vomer (the others refer to the bones of the middle ear)
55. Ulna (the others refer to the coxal bone)
56. Ethmoid (the others refer to the hand and wrist)
57. Nasal (the others refer to cranial bones)
58. Anvil (the others refer to the cervical vertebra)

Choose the Correct Term

59. a, p. 141
60. b, p. 141
61. b, p. 129
62. a, p. 141
63. b, p. 141

Matching

64. c, p. 131
65. g, p. 136
66. j, k, l, m, p. 140
67. n, p. 140
68. i, p. 138
69. a, p. 131
70. p, p. 140
71. b, d, p. 131
72. f, p. 131
73. h, q, p. 138
74. o, t, p. 140
75. r, p. 131
76. e, s, p. 131

Circle the Correct Answer

77. Diarthroses, p. 143
78. Synarthrotic, p. 143
79. Diarthrotic, p. 144
80. Ligaments, p. 145
81. Articular cartilage, p. 145
82. Least movable, p. 146
83. Largest, p. 144
84. 2, p. 145
85. Mobility, p. 146
86. Pivot, p. 145

Unscramble the Words

87. Vertebrae
88. Pubis
89. Scapula
90. Mandible
91. Phalanges
92. Pelvic girdle

Applying What You Know

93. The bones are responsible for the majority of our blood cell formation. The disease condition of the bones might be inhibiting the production of blood cells for Mrs. Perine.
94. Epiphyseal cartilage is present only while a child is still growing. It becomes bone in adulthood. It is particularly vulnerable to fractures in childhood and preadolescence.
95. Osteoporosis
96. Male bones are larger and have more distinct bumps and markings. Male bones also have greater tension on bones so the bones are bigger and denser at points of muscle attachment. Bones that have no epiphyseal plate have completed their growth and are adult bones.

97. WORD FIND

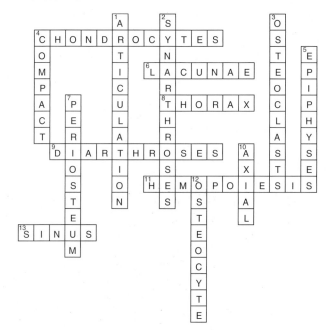

Matching

11. g, p. 143
12. b, p. 125
13. i, p. 125
14. j, p. 131
15. e, p. 136
16. h, p. 131
17. a, p. 138
18. c, p. 143
19. f, p. 145
20. d, p. 146

Longitudinal Section of Long Bone

1. Articular cartilage
2. Cancellous (spongy) bone
3. Epiphyseal line
4. Red marrow cavities
5. Compact bone
6. Medullary cavity
7. Endosteum
8. Yellow marrow
9. Periosteum
10. Epiphysis
11. Diaphysis

Crossword

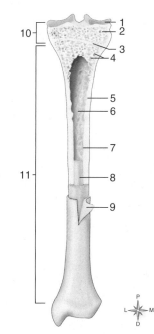

Check Your Knowledge

Multiple choice

1. a, p. 124
2. c, p. 124
3. a, p. 124
4. c, p. 136
5. c, p. 138
6. d, p. 125
7. c, p. 129
8. c, p. 135
9. d, p. 140 and Table 7-6
10. a, p. 143

Anterior View of Skeleton

1. Frontal bone
2. Nasal bone
3. Zygomatic bone
4. Sternum
5. Ribs
6. Vertebrae
7. Ilium
8. Pubis
9. Ischium
10. Greater trochanter
11. Phalanges
12. Metatarsals
13. Tarsals
14. Fibula
15. Tibia
16. Patella
17. Femur
18. Phalanges
19. Metacarpals
20. Carpals
21. Ulna
22. Radius
23. Humerus
24. Xiphoid process
25. Costal cartilage
26. Scapula
27. Manubrium
28. Clavicle
29. Mandible
30. Maxilla

Posterior View of Skeleton

1. Clavicle
2. Acromion process
3. Scapula
4. Ribs
5. Humerus
6. Ulna
7. Radius
8. Carpals
9. Metacarpals
10. Phalanges
11. Ilium
12. Ischium
13. Pubis
14. Coxal (hip) bone
15. Calcaneus (a tarsal bone)
16. Metatarsal bones
17. Phalanges
18. Tarsals
19. Fibula
20. Tibia
21. Femur
22. Sacrum
23. Lumbar vertebrae
24. Thoracic vertebrae
25. Cervical vertebrae
26. Occipital bone
27. Parietal bone

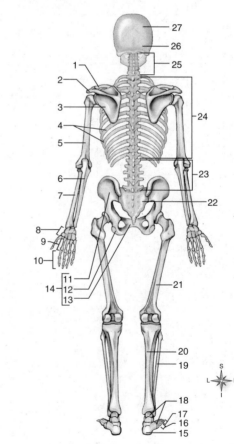

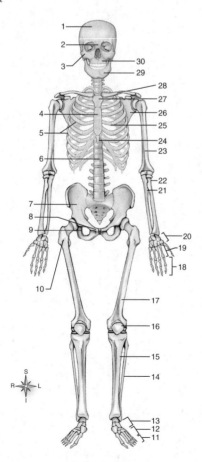

Skull Viewed from the Right Side

1. Parietal bone	9. Frontal bone
2. Squamous suture	10. Sphenoid bone
3. Occipital bone	11. Ethmoid bone
4. Lambdoidal suture	12. Nasal bone
5. Temporal bone	13. Zygomatic bone
6. External auditory canal	14. Maxilla
7. Mastoid process	15. Mandible
8. Coronal suture	

Structure of a Diarthrotic Joint

1. Bone
2. Periosteum
3. Blood vessel
4. Nerve
5. Articular cartilage
6. Joint cavity
7. Joint capsule
8. Articular cartilage
9. Synovial membrane

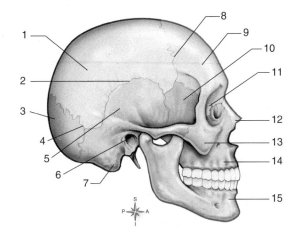

Skull Viewed from the Front

1. Sphenoid bone	7. Parietal bone
2. Ethmoid bone	8. Nasal bone
3. Lacrimal bone	9. Inferior concha
4. Zygomatic bone	10. Maxilla
5. Vomer	11. Mandible
6. Frontal bone	

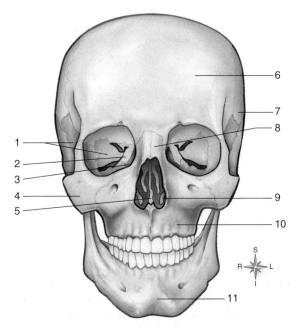

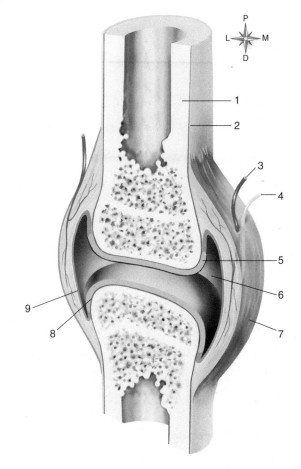

CHAPTER 8 MUSCULAR SYSTEM

Select the Correct Term

1. a, b, p. 156
2. b, p. 156
3. c, p. 156
4. c, p. 156
5. a, p. 156
6. b, p. 156
7. b, c, p. 156
8. a, p. 156
9. c, p. 156
10. c, p. 156

Matching

Group A

11. d, p. 156
12. b, p. 156
13. a, p. 156
14. e, p. 156
15. c, p. 156

Group B

16. e, p. 157
17. c, p. 157
18. b, p. 157
19. a, p. 157
20. d, p. 157

Fill in the Blanks

21. Pulling, p. 159
22. Insertion, p. 159
23. Insertion, origin, p. 159
24. Prime mover, p. 159
25. Antagonists, p. 159
26. Synergist, p. 160
27. Tonic contraction, p. 160
28. Muscle tone, p. 160
29. Hypothermia, p. 160
30. ATP, p. 160

True or False

31. Neuromuscular junction, not motor neuron, p. 161
32. T
33. T
34. Oxygen debt, not fatigue, p. 161
35. "All or none," not "must," p. 161
36. Lactic acid, not ATP, p. 161
37. T
38. T
39. Skeletal muscles, not smooth muscles, p. 161
40. T

Select the Correct Answer

41. a, p. 162
42. b, p. 162
43. b, p. 163
44. c, p. 163
45. d, p. 163
46. a, p. 161
47. b, p. 162
48. c, p. 162
49. b, p. 163
50. d, p. 163

Select the Correct Answer

51. a, p. 164
52. d, p. 164
53. c, p. 164
54. a, p. 164
55. d, p. 164
56. c, p. 165

Select the Best Choice or Choices

57. c, p. 168
58. a, d, f, pp. 166 and 168
59. b, f, pp. 166 and 168
60. a, p. 166
61. c, p. 166
62. b, f, pp. 166 and 168
63. a, p. 166
64. a, d, pp. 166 and 168
65. b, p. 166
66. b, p. 166
67. a, e, p. 168
68. b, p. 168
69. d, p. 168

Unscramble the Words

70. Flexion
71. Actin
72. Eversion
73. Origin
74. Sarcomere
75. Extension

Applying What You Know

76. Bursitis
77. (a) Carpal tunnel syndrome. (b) The wrist, hand, and fingers are affected due to tenosynovitis. Pain may radiate to the forearm and shoulder. (c) Injections of anti-inflammatory agents or surgical removal of tissue pressing on the median nerve.
78. Tendon
79. WORD FIND

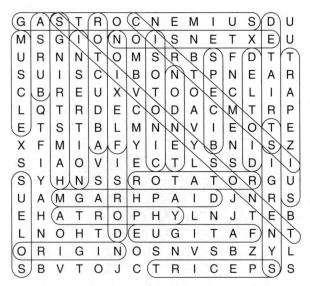

Crossword

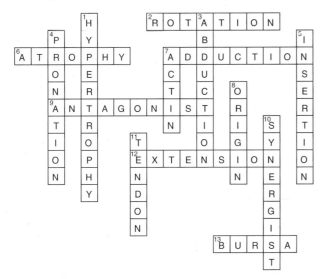

Muscles—Anterior View

1. Sternocleidomastoid
2. Trapezius
3. Pectoralis major
4. Rectus abdominis
5. External abdominal oblique
6. Iliopsoas
7. Quadriceps group
8. Tibialis anterior
9. Peroneus longus
10. Peroneus brevis
11. Soleus
12. Gastrocnemius
13. Sartorius
14. Adductor group
15. Brachialis
16. Biceps brachii
17. Deltoid
18. Facial muscles

Check Your Knowledge

Multiple Choice

1. d, p. 163
2. a, p. 164
3. c, p. 162
4. b, p. 161
5. a, p. 159
6. b, p. 157
7. d, p. 160
8. a, p. 156
9. a, p. 156
10. c, p. 171

True or False

11. T
12. T
13. Myosin, not actin, p. 157
14. Posterior, not anterior, p. 157
15. T
16. T
17. T
18. Flexion, not abduction, p. 164
19. T
20. T

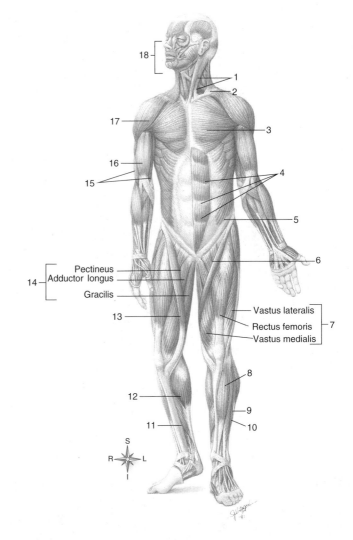

Muscles—Posterior View

1. Trapezius
2. External abdominal oblique
3. Gluteus maximus
4. Adductor magnus
5. Soleus
6. Peroneus brevis
7. Peroneus longus
8. Gastrocnemius
9. Hamstring group
10. Latissimus dorsi
11. Triceps brachii
12. Deltoid
13. Sternocleidomastoid

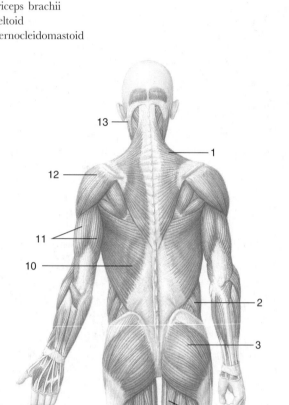

CHAPTER 9
NERVOUS SYSTEM

Matching

Group A

1. b, p. 179
2. c, p. 179
3. d, p. 179
4. a, p. 179

Group B

5. b, p. 179
6. d, p. 179
7. c, p. 181
8. a, p. 179
9. f, p. 182
10. e, p. 182

Select the Correct Term

11. a, p. 179
12. b, p. 181
13. b, p. 181
14. a, p. 181
15. a, p. 181
16. b, p. 181
17. b, p. 181
18. a, p. 181
19. b, p. 184
20. a, p. 179

Fill in the Blanks

21. Two-neuron arc, p. 182
22. Sensory, interneurons, and motor neurons, p. 183
23. Receptors, p. 183
24. Synapse, p. 185
25. Reflex, p. 183
26. Withdrawal reflex, p. 184
27. Ganglion, p. 183
28. Interneurons, p. 184
29. "Knee jerk," p. 183
30. Gray matter, p. 184

Circle the Correct Answer

31. Do not, p. 184
32. Increases, p. 184
33. Excess, p. 184
34. Postsynaptic, p. 187
35. Presynaptic, p. 187
36. Neurotransmitter, p. 187
37. Communicate, p. 187
38. Specifically, p. 187
39. Sleep, p. 187
40. Pain, p. 187

Select the Correct Answer

41. e, p. 188
42. d, p. 192
43. a, p. 188
44. e, p. 190
45. e, p. 190
46. d, p. 190

47. b, p. 190
48. e, p. 192
49. b, p. 192
50. d, p. 192
51. d, p. 189
52. b, p. 191
53. a, p. 192
54. d, p. 192
55. c, p. 190

True or False

56. 17-18 inches, not 24-25 inches, p. 193
57. Bottom of the first lumbar vertebra, not bottom of the sacrum, p. 193

58. Lumbar punctures, not CAT scans, p. 197
59. Spinal tracts, not dendrites, p. 193
60. T
61. One general function, not several functions, p. 193
62. Anesthesia, not paralysis, p. 193

Circle the One That Does Not Belong

63. Ventricles (the others refer to meninges)
64. CSF (the others refer to the arachnoid)
65. Pia mater (the others refer to the cerebrospinal fluid)
66. Choroid plexus (the others refer to the dura mater)
67. Brain tumor (the others refer to a lumbar puncture)

68. Fill in the missing areas on the chart below.

Nerve		Conduct Impulses	Function
I	Olfactory		
II			Vision
III		From brain to eye muscles	
IV	Trochlear		
V			Sensations of face, scalp, and teeth, chewing movements
VI		From brain to external eye muscles	
VII			Sense of taste, contractions of muscles of facial expression
VIII	Vestibulocochlear		
IX		From throat and taste buds of tongue to brain, also from brain to throat muscles and salivary glands	
X	Vagus		
XI			Shoulder movements, turning movements of head
XII	Hypoglossal		

Select the Correct Term

69. a, p. 197
70. b, p. 199
71. a, p. 197
72. b, p. 203
73. b, p. 197
74. a, p. 198
75. b, p. 197
76. b, p. 197

Matching

77. d, p. 199
78. e, p. 200
79. f, p. 200
80. b, p. 200
81. a, p. 199
82. c, p. 199

Select the Correct Answer

83. c, p. 201
84. b, p. 201
85. b, p. 201
86. d, p. 201
87. a, p. 201
88. a, p. 202

Select the Correct Term

89. b, p. 202
90. a, p. 202
91. a, p. 202
92. b, p. 202
93. a, p. 202
94. b, p. 202
95. a, p. 202
96. a, p. 202
97. b, p. 202
98. b, p. 202

Fill in the Blanks

99. Acetylcholine, p. 202
100. Adrenergic fibers, p. 202
101. Cholinergic fibers, p. 202
102. Homeostasis, p. 202
103. Heart rate, p. 202
104. Decreased, p. 204

Unscramble the Words

105. Neurons
106. Synapse
107. Autonomic
108. Smooth muscle
109. Sympathetic

Applying What You Know

110. Right
111. Hydrocephalus
112. Sympathetic
113. Parasympathetic
114. Sympathetic; no, the digestive process is not active during sympathetic control. Bill may experience nausea, vomiting, or discomfort because of this factor. See p. 202.
115. WORD FIND

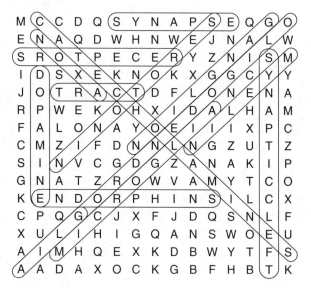

Crossword

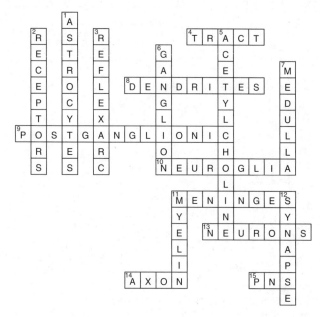

Check Your Knowledge

Multiple Choice

1. d, p. 181
2. b, p. 179
3. a, p. 181
4. b, p. 182
5. a, p. 183
6. d, p. 187
7. d, p. 188
8. c, p. 190
9. c, p. 194
10. d, p. 199

Matching

11. c, p. 184
12. a, p. 190
13. j, p. 192
14. h, p. 195
15. b, p. 198
16. i, p. 197
17. f, p. 200
18. e, p. 201
19. d, p. 202
20. g, p. 192

Neurons

1. Dendrites
2. Cell body
3. Mitochondrion
4. Nucleus
5. Axon
6. Schwann cell
7. Node of Ranvier
8. Nucleus of Schwann cell
9. Myelin sheath
10. Axon
11. Cell membrane of axon
12. Neurilemma (sheath of Schwann cell)

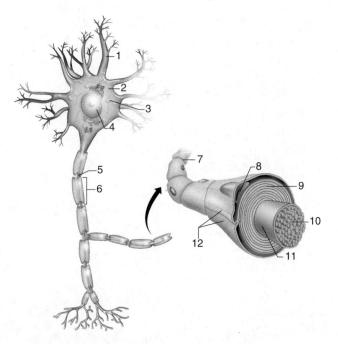

Cranial Nerves

1. Olfactory nerve
2. Trigeminal nerve
3. Glossopharyngeal nerve
4. Hypoglossal nerve
5. Accessory nerve
6. Vagus nerve
7. Vestibulocochlear nerve
8. Facial nerve
9. Abducens nerve
10. Oculomotor nerve
11. Optic nerve
12. Trochlear nerve

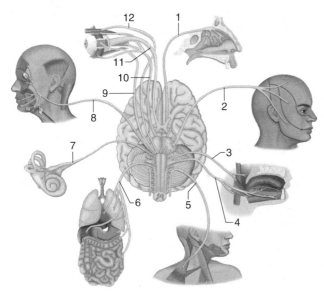

The Cerebrum

1. Occipital lobe
2. Temporal lobe
3. Lateral fissure
4. Frontal lobe
5. Central sulcus
6. Parietal lobe

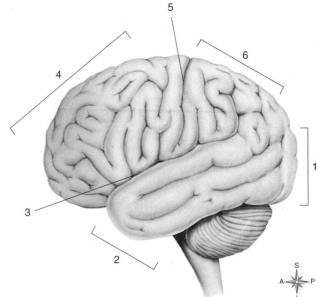

Neural Pathway Involved in the Patellar Reflex

1. Dorsal root ganglion
2. Sensory neuron
3. Stretch receptor
4. Patella
5. Patellar tendon
6. Quadriceps muscle
7. Motor neuron
8. Monosynaptic synapse
9. Gray matter
10. Interneuron

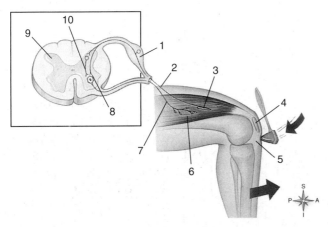

Sagittal Section of the Central Nervous System

1. Skull
2. Pineal gland
3. Cerebellum
4. Midbrain
5. Spinal cord
6. Medulla
7. Reticular formation
8. Pons
9. Pituitary gland
10. Hypothalamus
11. Cerebral cortex
12. Thalamus
13. Corpus callosum

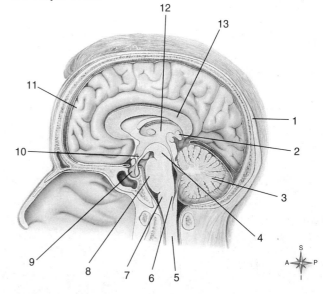

Autonomic Conduction Paths

1. Axon of somatic motor neuron
2. Cell body of somatic motor neuron
3. Spinal cord
4. Gray matter
5. Cell body of preganglionic neuron
6. Dorsal root
7. Ventral root
8. Axon of preganglionic sympathetic neuron
9. Axon of postganglionic neuron
10. Sympathetic ganglion
11. Collateral ganglion
12. Axon of postganglionic sympathetic neuron

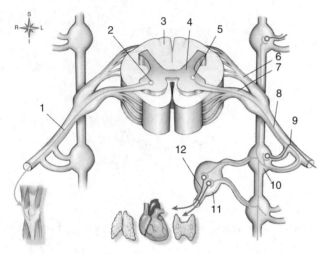

CHAPTER 10 SENSES

Matching

1. d, pp. 214-215
2. b, p. 214
3. a, p. 215
4. e, p. 214
5. c, p. 215
6. d, p. 215
7. c, p. 214
8. e, p. 216
9. a, p. 216
10. b, p. 214

Select the Correct Answer

11. c, p. 217
12. e, p. 217
13. b, p. 217
14. c, p. 217
15. e, p. 217
16. d, p. 218
17. a, p. 218
18. b, p. 218
19. c, p. 221
20. b, p. 221
21. d, p. 219
22. a, p. 220
23. d, p. 221

Select the Correct Term

24. b, p. 222
25. c, p. 223
26. b, p. 222
27. a, p. 222
28. c, p. 223
29. a, p. 222
30. c, p. 223
31. b, p. 222
32. b, p. 222
33. c, p. 224

Fill in the Blanks

34. Auricle; external auditory canal, p. 222
35. Eardrum, p. 222
36. Ossicles, p. 222
37. Oval window, p. 222
38. Otitis media, p. 223
39. Vestibule, p. 223
40. Mechanoreceptors, p. 224
41. Crista ampullaris, p. 226

Circle the Correct Answer

42. Papillae, p. 226
43. Cranial, p. 226
44. Mucus, p. 227
45. Memory, p. 227
46. Chemoreceptors, pp. 215-216

Unscramble the Words

47. Auricle
48. Sclera
49. Papilla
50. Conjunctiva
51. Pupils

Applying What You Know

52. External otitis
53. Cataracts
54. The eustachian tube connects the throat to the middle ear and provides a perfect pathway for the spread of infection.
55. Olfactory
56. WORD FIND

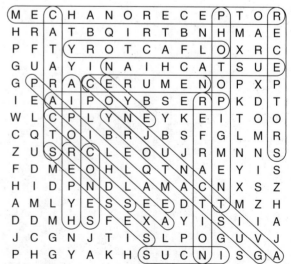

Crossword

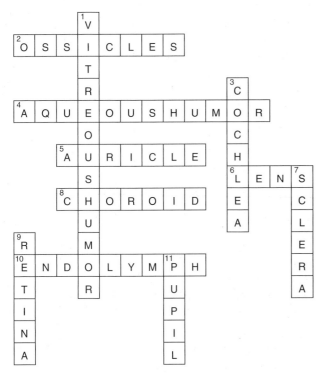

1. V
2. OSSICLES
3. C (VTR...)
4. AQUEOUSHUMOR
5. AURICLE
6. LENS
8. CHOROID
9. R
10. ENDOLYMPH
11. PUPIL

(Crossword grid letters: V / OSSICLES / T / R / C / AQUEOUSHUMOR / E O S / AURICLE / C H O / S R / CHOROID / E A / U C / R L / RETINA / ENDOLYMPH / R U P I L / S C L E R A)

Eye

1. Pupil
2. Lens
3. Lacrimal caruncle
4. Sclera
5. Choroid
6. Retina
7. Optic disk
8. Optic nerve
9. Central artery and vein
10. Macula
11. Fovea
12. Posterior chamber
13. Fibrous layer
14. Vascular layer
15. Inner layer
16. Ciliary muscle
17. Lower lid
18. Iris
19. Anterior chamber
20. Cornea

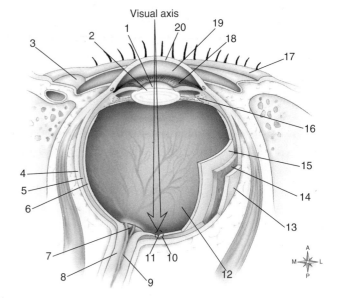

Visual axis

Check Your Knowledge

Multiple Choice

1. a, p. 215
2. b, p. 221
3. a, p. 222
4. c, p. 221
5. b, p. 222
6. b, p. 223
7. d, p. 216
8. b, p. 221
9. d, p. 222
10. a, p. 220

True or False

11. T
12. Window of the eye, not white of the eye, p. 216
13. T
14. Cataract, not glaucoma, p. 219
15. T
16. T
17. T
18. T
19. T
20. T

Ear

1. Auricle
2. Temporal bone
3. External auditory meatus
4. Tympanic membrane
5. Semicircular canals
6. Oval window
7. Facial nerve
8. Vestibular nerve
9. Cochlear nerve
10. Cochlea
11. Vestibule
12. Auditory tube
13. Stapes
14. Incus
15. Malleus

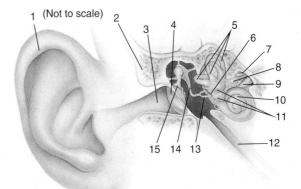

(Not to scale)

CHAPTER 11
ENDOCRINE SYSTEM

Matching

Group A

1. d, p. 238
2. c, p. 238
3. e, p. 238
4. a, p. 238
5. b, p. 238

Group B

6. e, p. 239
7. c, p. 241
8. a, p. 239
9. d, p. 238
10. b, p. 238

Fill in the Blanks

11. First messengers, p. 238
12. Endocrine glands, p. 238
13. Target organs, p. 238
14. Cyclic AMP, p. 239
15. Second messenger, p. 239
16. Communication, p. 239
17. Target cells, p. 239

Select the Correct Answer

18. b, p. 242
19. e, p. 244
20. d, p. 240
21. d, p. 240
22. a, p. 243
23. c, p. 244
24. c, p. 244
25. b, p. 243
26. a, p. 243
27. a, p. 243
28. d, p. 244
29. b, p. 244
30. a, p. 244
31. c, p. 245
32. c, p. 245

Select the Correct Term

33. a, p. 242
34. b, p. 244
35. b, p. 245
36. c, p. 245
37. a, p. 243
38. c, p. 245
39. a, p. 243
40. a, p. 243
41. a, p. 243
42. c, p. 245

Circle the Correct Answer

43. Below, p. 245
44. Calcitonin, p. 246
45. Iodine, p. 246
46. Do not, p. 246
47. Thyroid, p. 246
48. Decrease, p. 247
49. Hypothyroidism, p. 246
50. Cretinism, p. 246
51. PTH, p. 247
52. Increase, p. 247

Fill in the Blanks

53. Adrenal cortex; adrenal medulla, p. 247
54. Corticoids, p. 248
55. Mineralocorticoids, p. 248
56. Glucocorticoids, p. 248
57. Sex hormones, p. 248
58. Gluconeogenesis, p. 248
59. Blood pressure, p. 248
60. Epinephrine; norepinephrine, p. 249
61. Stress, p. 250
62. Addison disease, p. 250

Select the Correct Term

63. a, p. 248
64. a, p. 248
65. b, p. 249
66. a, p. 250
67. b, p. 250
68. a, p. 248
69. a, p. 249

Circle the Term That Does Not Belong

70. Beta cells (the others refer to glucagon)
71. Glucagon (the others refer to insulin)
72. Thymosin (the others refer to female sex glands)
73. Chorion (the others refer to male sex glands)
74. Aldosterone (the others refer to the thymus)
75. ACTH (the others refer to the placenta)
76. Semen (the others refer to the pineal gland)

Matching

Group A

77. e, p. 250
78. c, p. 250
79. b, p. 253
80. d, p. 253
81. a, p. 252

Group B

82. e, p. 253
83. a, p. 253
84. b, p. 253
85. c, p. 253
86. d, p. 253

True or False

87. T
88. T
89. Leptin, not ghrelin, p. 253
90. T
91. Ghrelin, not leptin, p. 253

Unscramble the Words

92. Corticoids
93. Diuresis
94. Glucocorticoids
95. Steroids
96. Stress

Applying What You Know

97. She was pregnant.
98. Adrenal cortex; this source of testosterone may produce secondary male characteristics if unattended to at this young age.
99. Oxytocin

100. WORD FIND

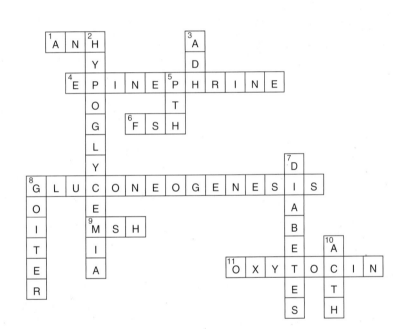

Crossword

Check Your Knowledge

Multiple Choice

1. a, p. 237
2. c, p. 243
3. d, p. 241
4. c, p. 244
5. d, p. 251
6. d, p. 245
7. b, p. 246
8. d, p. 250
9. d, p. 253
10. b, p. 253

Matching

11. j, p. 239
12. g, p. 241
13. h, p. 243
14. i, p. 246
15. b, p. 248
16. f, p. 248
17. a, p. 250
18. d, p. 252
19. e, p. 253
20. c, p. 253

Endocrine Glands

1. Pineal
2. Hypothalamus
3. Pituitary
4. Thyroid
5. Thymus
6. Adrenals
7. Pancreas islets
8. Ovaries (female)
9. Testes (male)
10. Parathyroids

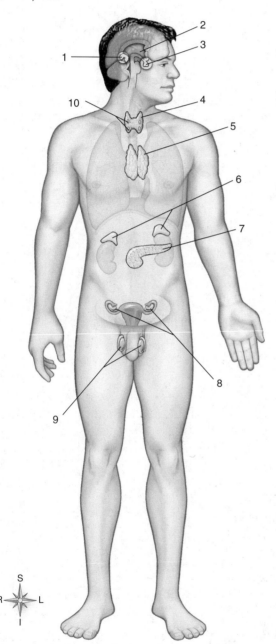

CHAPTER 12
BLOOD

Select the Correct Answer

1. e, p. 264
2. d, p. 264
3. d, p. 265
4. b, p. 265
5. c, p. 265
6. a, p. 268
7. b, p. 266
8. d, p. 265
9. c, p. 265
10. d, p. 267
11. a, p. 268
12. b, p. 268
13. b, p. 265
14. b, p. 265
15. e, p. 266
16. b, p. 265
17. c, p. 265
18. d, p. 266
19. d, p. 267
20. d, p. 267
21. Fill in the missing areas.

Blood Type	Antigen	Antibody
A	A	
B		Anti-A
AB	A, B	
O		Anti-A, Anti-B

Fill in the Blanks

22. Antigen, p. 269
23. Antibody, p. 269
24. Agglutinate, p. 269
25. Erythroblastosis fetalis, p. 271
26. Rhesus monkey, p. 270
27. RhoGAM, p. 271
28. AB positive, p. 271

Select the Correct Answer

29. b, p. 272
30. b, p. 272
31. c, p. 273
32. b, p. 273
33. a, p. 273
34. e, p. 273
35. a, p. 273
36. d, p. 273
37. e, p. 273
38. b, p. 273
39. c, p. 274

Circle the Correct Response

40. Hemorrhagic stroke, p. 274
41. 0.8, p. 274
42. Thrombus, p. 273
43. Low-dose aspirin, p. 274
44. Anticoagulant drugs, p. 274
45. Phlebotomist, p. 276

Unscramble the Words

46. Phagocyte
47. Thrombin
48. Antigen
49. Fibrin
50. Typing

Applying What You Know

51. No. If Mrs. Lassiter had a negative Rh factor and her husband had a positive Rh factor, it would set up the strong possibility of erythroblastosis fetalis.
52. Both procedures assist the clotting process.
53. WORD FIND

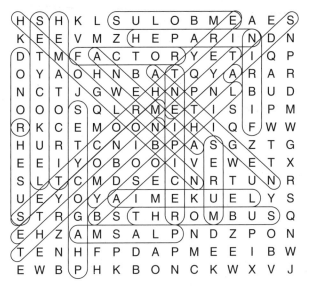

Crossword

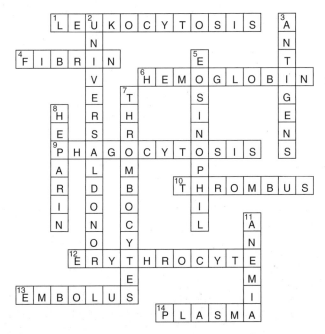

Check Your Knowledge

Multiple Choice

1. b, p. 263
2. b, p. 265
3. a, p. 265
4. a, p. 267
5. d, p. 274
6. a, p. 273
7. a, p. 273
8. d, p. 269
9. c, p. 271
10. b, p. 271

Matching

11. d, p. 264
12. f, p. 265
13. h, p. 265
14. a, p. 266
15. g, p. 267
16. c, p. 272
17. b, p. 272
18. e, p. 268
19. i, p. 272
20. j, p. 271

Human Blood Cells

BODY CELL		FUNCTION
Erythrocyte		Oxygen and carbon dioxide transport
Neutrophil		Immune defense (phagocytosis)
Eosinophil		Defense against parasites
Basophil		Inflammatory response and heparin secretion
B lymphocyte		Antibody production (precursor of plasma cells)
T lymphocyte		Cellular immune response
Monocyte		Immune defenses (phagocytosis)
Thrombocyte		Blood clotting

Blood Typing

Recipient's blood		Reactions with donor's blood			
RBC antigens	Plasma antibodies	Donor type O	Donor type A	Donor type B	Donor type AB
None (Type O)	Anti-A Anti-B				
A (Type A)	Anti-B				
B (Type B)	Anti-A				
AB (Type AB)	(none)				

Normal blood   Agglutinated blood

CHAPTER 13
CARDIOVASCULAR SYSTEM

Fill in the Blanks

1. CPR, p. 285
2. Interatrial septum, p. 285
3. Atria, p. 285
4. Ventricles, p. 285
5. Myocardium, p. 285
6. Endocarditis, p. 285
7. Bicuspid or mitral; tricuspid, p. 286
8. Pulmonary circulation, p. 287
9. Coronary embolism or coronary thrombosis, p. 288
10. Myocardial infarction, p. 288
11. Sinoatrial, p. 291
12. P; QRS complex; T, p. 292
13. Repolarization, p. 292

Choose the Correct Term

14. a, p. 286
15. k, p. 285
16. g, p. 287
17. c, p. 285
18. d, p. 286
19. f, p. 285
20. h, p. 288
21. b, p. 288
22. e, p. 291
23. i, p. 286
24. j, p. 292
25. l, p. 284
26. m, p. 286

Circle the Correct Answer

27. Per minute, p. 292
28. Parasympathetic, p. 292
29. Higher, p. 293
30. Contraction, p. 293
31. 5, p. 292

Matching

32. d, p. 294
33. b, p. 294
34. c, p. 294
35. g, p. 294
36. a, p. 295
37. e, p. 294
38. f, p. 294

Multiple Choice

39. d, p. 299
40. c, p. 299
41. b, p. 296
42. a, p. 294
43. b, p. 296
44. b, p. 299
45. d, p. 301
46. b, p. 302
47. b, p. 302
48. a, p. 302
49. d, p. 294
50. a, p. 295

True or False

51. Highest in arteries, lowest in veins, p. 302
52. Blood pressure gradient, not deficit, p. 302
53. Stop, not increase, p. 303
54. High blood pressure, not low, p. 303
55. Decreases, not increases, p. 303
56. T
57. T
58. T
59. Stronger will increase, weaker will decrease, p. 304
60. Contract, not relax, p. 306
61. Relax, not contract, p. 306
62. Artery, not vein, p. 306
63. T
64. T
65. Brachial, not dorsalis pedis, p. 307

Unscramble the Words

66. Systemic
67. Venule
68. Artery
69. Pulse
70. Vessel

Applying What You Know

71. Coronary bypass surgery
72. Artificial pacemaker
73. The endocardial lining can become rough and abrasive to red blood cells passing over its surface. As a result, a fatal blood clot may be formed.
74. Dan may be hemorrhaging. The heart beats faster during hemorrhage in an attempt to compensate for blood loss.

75. WORD FIND

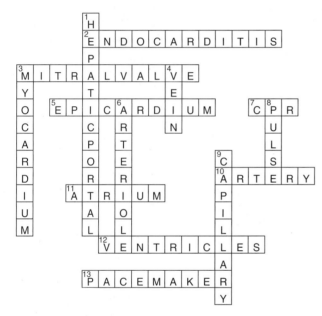

Crossword

[Crossword grid with the following filled answers:]

2. ENDOCARDITIS
3. MITRALVALVE
5. EPICARDIUM
7. CPR
10. ARTERY
11. ATRIUM
12. VENTRICLES
13. PACEMAKER

[Down answers visible: HEP (1), MYOCARDIUM (3), VEIN (4), CARTER (6), PULS (8), CAPILLARY (9)]

Check Your Knowledge

Multiple Choice

1. a, p. 284
2. c, p. 286
3. b, p. 286
4. a, p. 291
5. a, p. 294
6. d, p. 291
7. c, p. 303
8. d, p. 308
9. c, p. 293
10. c, p. 295

Matching

11. f, p. 285
12. g, p. 285
13. h, p. 286
14. i, p. 286
15. j, p. 297
16. b, p. 291
17. c, p. 285
18. a, p. 306
19. d, p. 307
20. e, p. 286

The Heart

1. Left common carotid artery
2. Left subclavian artery
3. Arch of aorta
4. Left pulmonary artery
5. Left atrium
6. Left pulmonary veins
7. Great cardiac vein
8. Branches of left coronary artery and cardiac vein
9. Left ventricle
10. Apex
11. Right ventricle
12. Right atrium
13. Right coronary artery and cardiac vein
14. Right pulmonary veins
15. Ascending aorta
16. Right pulmonary artery
17. Superior vena cava
18. Brachiocephalic trunk

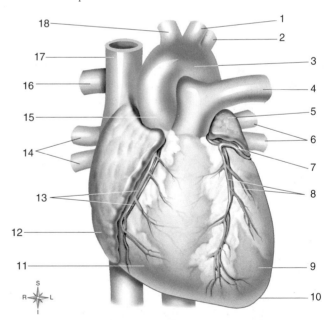

Conduction System of the Heart

1. Atrioventricular (AV) node
2. Sinoatrial (SA) node (pacemaker)
3. Internodal bundles
4. AV bundle (of His)
5. Lateral ventricular wall
6. Septum
7. Right and left branches of AV bundle (bundle of His)
8. Subendocardial fibers (Purkinje fibers)
9. Interatrial bundle

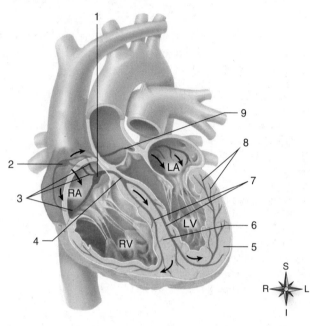

Fetal Circulation

1. Aortic arch
2. Abdominal aorta
3. Common iliac artery
4. Internal iliac arteries
5. Umbilical arteries
6. Fetal umbilicus
7. Umbilical cord
8. Fetal side of placenta
9. Maternal side of placenta
10. Umbilical vein
11. Hepatic portal vein
12. Ductus venosus
13. Inferior vena cava
14. Foramen ovale
15. Superior vena cava
16. Ascending aorta
17. Pulmonary trunk
18. Ductus arteriosus

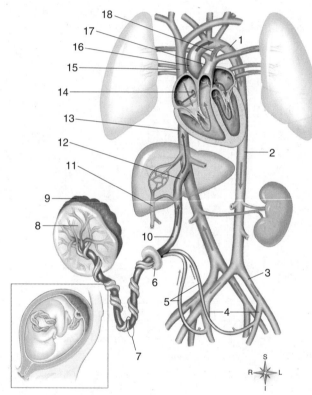

Hepatic Portal Circulation

1. Inferior vena cava
2. Stomach
3. Gastric vein
4. Spleen
5. Pancreatic vein
6. Splenic vein
7. Gastroepiploic vein
8. Descending colon
9. Inferior mesenteric vein
10. Small intestine
11. Appendix
12. Ascending colon
13. Superior mesenteric vein
14. Pancreas
15. Duodenum
16. Hepatic portal vein
17. Liver
18. Hepatic veins

Principal Arteries of the Body

1. Right common carotid
2. Brachiocephalic
3. Right coronary
4. Axillary
5. Brachial
6. Superior mesenteric
7. Abdominal aorta
8. Common iliac
9. Internal iliac
10. External iliac
11. Deep femoral
12. Femoral
13. Popliteal
14. Anterior tibial
15. Occipital
16. Facial
17. Internal carotid
18. External carotid
19. Left common carotid
20. Left subclavian
21. Arch of aorta
22. Pulmonary
23. Left coronary
24. Aorta
25. Splenic
26. Renal
27. Celiac
28. Inferior mesenteric
29. Radial
30. Ulnar

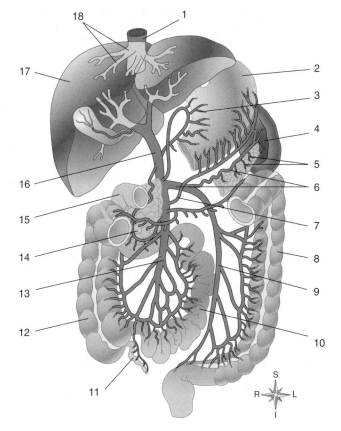

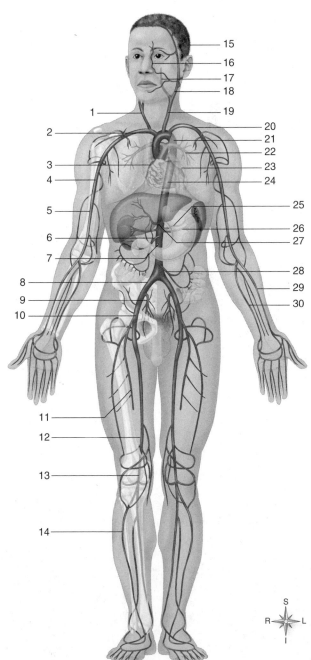

Principal Veins of the Body

1. Right brachiocephalic
2. Right subclavian
3. Superior vena cava
4. Right pulmonary
5. Small cardiac
6. Inferior vena cava
7. Hepatic
8. Hepatic portal
9. Superior mesenteric
10. Median cubital
11. Common iliac
12. External iliac
13. Femoral
14. Great saphenous
15. Fibular (peroneal)
16. Anterior tibial
17. Posterior tibial
18. Occipital
19. Facial
20. External jugular
21. Internal jugular
22. Left brachiocephalic
23. Left subclavian
24. Axillary
25. Cephalic
26. Great cardiac
27. Basilic
28. Brachial veins
29. Long thoracic
30. Splenic
31. Inferior mesenteric
32. Ulnar vein
33. Radial vein
34. Common iliac
35. Internal iliac
36. Digital veins
37. Femoral
38. Popliteal

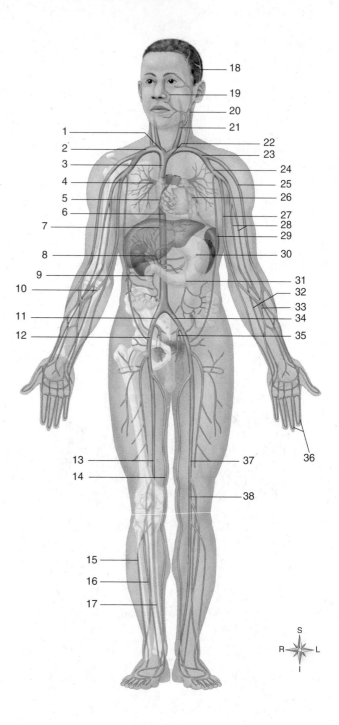

Normal ECG Deflections

1. Atrial depolarization
2. Ventricular depolarization
3. Ventricular repolarization

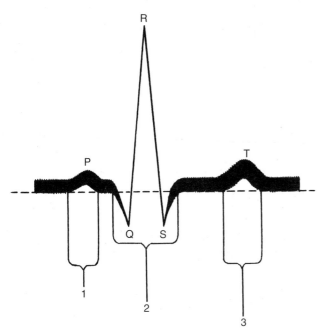

CHAPTER 14
LYMPHATIC SYSTEM AND IMMUNITY

Fill in the Blanks

1. Lymph, p. 318
2. Interstitial fluid, p. 319
3. Lymphatic capillaries, p. 319
4. Right lymphatic duct; thoracic duct, p. 320
5. Cisterna chyli, p. 320
6. Lymph nodes, p. 320
7. Afferent, p. 320
8. Efferent, p. 320

Select the Correct Term

9. b, p. 322
10. c, p. 322
11. c, p. 322
12. a, p. 321
13. c, p. 322
14. a, p. 321
15. a, p. 321

Matching

16. c, p. 322
17. a, p. 325
18. e, p. 324
19. b, p. 325
20. d, p. 324

Choose the Correct Term

21. c, p. 328
22. d, p. 328
23. e, p. 325
24. a, p. 326
25. h, p. 326
26. b, p. 326
27. i, p. 326
28. f, p. 327
29. j, p. 326
30. g, p. 327

Circle the One That Does Not Belong

31. Allergy (the others refer to antibodies)
32. Fever (the others refer to antigens)
33. Memory (the others refer to nonspecific immunity)
34. Complement (the others refer to allergy)
35. Macrophage (the others refer to complement)

Multiple Choice

36. d, p. 329
37. d, p. 329
38. c, p. 330
39. b, p. 323
40. c, p. 329
41. c, p. 329
42. e, p. 329
43. e, p. 330
44. c, p. 330
45. e, p. 330
46. e, p. 330
47. d, p. 333
48. e, p. 326
49. a, p. 330
50. b, p. 330

Fill in the Blanks

51. Stem cell, p. 329
52. Liver and bone marrow; bone marrow, p. 329
53. Plasma cells, p. 330
54. Thymus gland, p. 330
55. Azidothymidine (AZT), p. 333
56. AIDS, p. 333
57. Vaccine, p. 333

Unscramble the Words

58. Complement
59. Immunity
60. Clones
61. Interferon
62. Memory cells

Applying What You Know

63. Interferon would possibly decrease the severity of the chickenpox virus.
64. AIDS
65. Baby Phelps had no means of producing T cells, thus making him susceptible to several diseases. Isolation is a means of controlling his exposure to these diseases.

66. WORD FIND

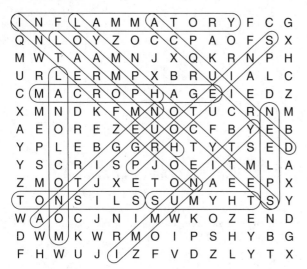

Crossword

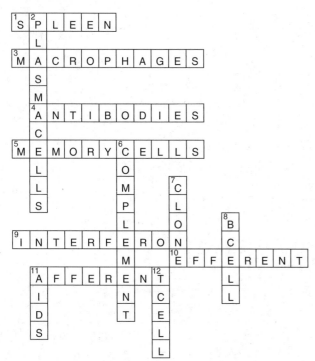

Check Your Knowledge

Multiple Choice

1. a, p. 319
2. a, p. 322
3. d, p. 320
4. b, p. 320
5. d, p. 321
6. b, p. 322
7. d, p. 325
8. d, p. 330
9. d, p. 323
10. c, p. 326

Matching

11. e, p. 320
12. d, p. 321
13. i, p. 323
14. h, p. 323
15. g, p. 326
16. b, p. 328
17. a, p. 326
18. j, p. 325
19. c, p. 326
20. f, p. 328

Principal Organs of the Lymphatic System

1. Tonsils
2. Submandibular nodes
3. Axillary lymph nodes
4. Thymus
5. Thoracic duct
6. Spleen
7. Cisterna chyli
8. Inguinal lymph nodes
9. Popliteal lymph nodes
10. Lymph vessels
11. Red bone marrow
12. Right lymphatic duct
13. Cervical lymph nodes

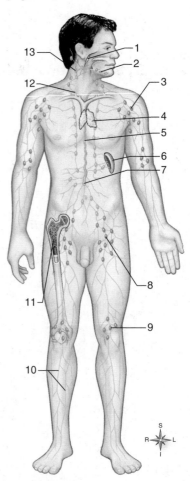

CHAPTER 15
RESPIRATORY SYSTEM

Matching

1. j, p. 343
2. g, p. 343
3. a, p. 342
4. i, p. 343
5. b, p. 344
6. f, p. 343
7. c, p. 342
8. h, p. 343
9. d, p. 343
10. e, p. 341

Fill in the Blanks

11. Air distributor, p. 342
12. Gas exchanger, p. 342
13. Filters, p. 341
14. Warms, p. 341
15. Humidifies, p. 341
16. Nose, p. 342
17. Pharynx, p. 342
18. Larynx, p. 342
19. Trachea, p. 342
20. Bronchi, p. 342
21. Lungs, p. 342
22. Alveoli, p. 342
23. Diffusion, p. 342
24. Respiratory mucosa, p. 343
25. Goblet, p. 343

Circle the One That Does Not Belong

26. Oropharynx (the others refer to the nose)
27. Conchae (the others refer to the paranasal sinuses)
28. Epiglottis (the others refer to the pharynx)
29. Uvula (the others refer to the adenoids)
30. Larynx (the others refer to the eustachian tubes)
31. Tonsils (the others refer to the larynx)
32. Eustachian tube (the others refer to the tonsils)
33. Pharynx (the others refer to the larynx)

Choose the Correct Term

34. a, p. 344
35. b, p. 344
36. a, p. 344
37. a, p. 344
38. a, p. 344
39. b, p. 345
40. b, p. 345
41. c, p. 345

Fill in the Blanks

42. Trachea, p. 346
43. Cartilage (C-rings), p. 346
44. Suffocation, p. 346
45. Primary bronchi, p. 348
46. Alveolar sacs, p. 348
47. Apex, p. 349
48. Pleura, p. 349
49. Pleurisy, p. 349
50. Pneumothorax, p. 349

True or False

51. Breathing, not diffusion, p. 352
52. Expiration, not inspiration, p. 353
53. Down, not up, p. 352 (review Chapter 3)
54. Internal, not external respiration, p. 351
55. T
56. 1 pint, not 2 pints, p. 353
57. T
58. Vital capacity, not residual volume, p. 353
59. T

Multiple Choice

60. e, p. 351
61. c, p. 359
62. c, p. 358
63. b, p. 353
64. d, p. 353
65. d, p. 353
66. d, p. 353

Matching

67. e, p. 354
68. b, p. 355
69. g, p. 356
70. a, p. 356
71. f, p. 356
72. d, p. 356
73. c, p. 356

Unscramble the Words

74. Pleurisy
75. Bronchitis
76. Epistaxis
77. Adenoids
78. Inspiration

Applying What You Know

79. During the day Mr. Gorski's cilia are paralyzed because of his heavy smoking. They use the time when Mr. Gorski is asleep to sweep accumulations of mucus and bacteria toward the pharynx. When he awakes, these collections are waiting to be eliminated.
80. Swelling of the tonsils or adenoids caused by infection may make it difficult or impossible for air to travel from the nose into the throat. The individual may be forced to breathe through the mouth.

81. WORD FIND

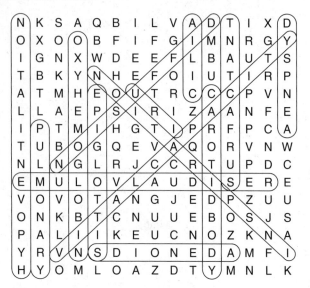

Crossword

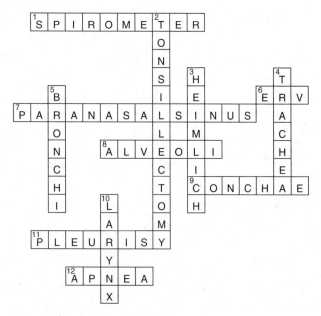

Check Your Knowledge

Multiple Choice

1. a, p. 342
2. b, p. 344
3. d, p. 341
4. b, p. 348
5. a, p. 353
6. d, p. 349
7. a, p. 351
8. c, p. 354
9. d, p. 356
10. b, p. 354

Matching

11. e, p. 343
12. i, p. 343
13. a, p. 344
14. g, p. 345

15. d, p. 346
16. b, p. 353
17. c, p. 355
18. h, p. 356
19. f, p. 356
20. j, p. 349

Sagittal View of the Head and Neck

1. Sphenoidal air sinus
2. Pharyngeal tonsil (adenoids)
3. Opening of auditory (eustachian) tube
4. Nasopharynx
5. Soft palate
6. Uvula
7. Palatine tonsil
8. Oropharynx
9. Epiglottis (part of larynx)
10. Laryngopharynx
11. Esophagus
12. Trachea
13. Vocal cords (part of larynx)
14. Thyroid cartilage (part of larynx)
15. Hyoid bone
16. Lingual tonsil
17. Hard palate
18. Inferior concha
19. Middle nasal concha of ethmoid
20. Superior nasal concha of ethmoid
21. Nasal bone
22. Frontal sinus

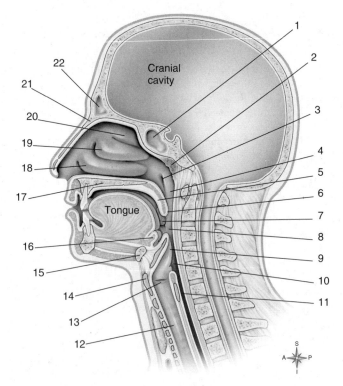

Respiratory Organs

1. Nasal cavity
2. Nasopharynx
3. Oropharynx
4. Laryngopharynx
5. Pharynx
6. Larynx
7. Trachea
8. Bronchioles
9. Left and right primary bronchi
10. Alveolar duct
11. Alveolar sac
12. Pulmonary capillary
13. Alveoli

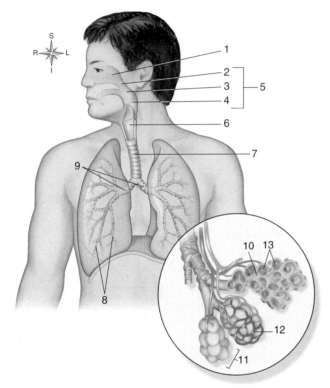

Pulmonary Ventilation Volumes

1. Total lung capacity
2. Inspiratory reserve volume
3. Tidal volume
4. Expiratory reserve volume
5. Residual volume
6. Vital capacity

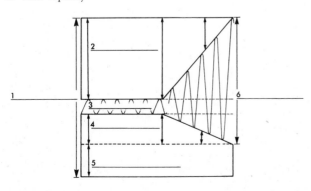

CHAPTER 16
DIGESTIVE SYSTEM

Fill in the Blanks

1. Gastrointestinal (GI) tract, p. 368
2. Mechanical, p. 368
3. Chemical, p. 369
4. Feces, p. 369
5. Digestion, p. 368
6. Absorption, p. 369
7. Mouth; anus, p. 369
8. Lumen, p. 369
9. Mucosa, p. 369
10. Submucosa, p. 370
11. Peristalsis, p. 370
12. Serosa, p. 370
13. Mesentery, p. 370

Choose the Correct Term

14. a, p. 368
15. b, p. 368
16. b, p. 368
17. a, p. 368
18. a, p. 368
19. a, p. 368
20. a, p. 368
21. a, p. 368
22. b, p. 368
23. b, p. 368
24. b, p. 368
25. b, p. 368

Select the Correct Answer

26. e, p. 370
27. c, p. 370
28. e, p. 372
29. d, p. 371
30. b, p. 371
31. c, p. 371
32. d, p. 372
33. d, p. 372
34. d, p. 372
35. a, p. 373
36. c, p. 372
37. a, p. 373
38. a, p. 372
39. b, p. 372
40. c, p. 373

Fill in the Blanks

41. Pharynx, p. 373
42. Esophagus, p. 374
43. Stomach, p. 374
44. Cardiac sphincter, or lower esophageal sphincter (LES), p. 374
45. Chyme, p. 375
46. Fundus, p. 375
47. Body, p. 375
48. Pylorus, p. 375
49. Pyloric sphincter, p. 376
50. Small intestine, p. 376

Matching

51. d, p. 375
52. j, p. 375
53. g, p. 375
54. a, p. 374
55. h, p. 376
56. b, p. 375
57. c, p. 375
58. e, p. 378
59. i, p. 376
60. f, p. 375

Select the Correct Answer

61. c, p. 376
62. b, p. 377
63. a, p. 379
64. a, p. 379
65. b, p. 378
66. e, p. 376
67. d, p. 378
68. d, p. 379; review Chapter 11 (hormones circulate in blood)
69. b, p. 379
70. c, p. 379

True or False

71. Vitamin K, not vitamin E, p. 382
72. No villi are present in the large intestine, p. 382
73. Diarrhea, not constipation, p. 382
74. Cecum, not sigmoid colon, p. 381
75. Hepatic, not splenic flexure, p. 381
76. Sigmoid, not splenic colon, p. 381
77. T
78. T
79. Parietal, not visceral, p. 383
80. Mesentery, not greater omentum, p. 383

Select the Correct Answer

81. b, p. 385
82. d, p. 384
83. c, p. 384
84. c, p. 384
85. c, p. 385

86. Fill in the blank areas on the chart below.

Digestive Juices and Enzymes	Substance Digested (or Hydrolyzed)	Resulting Product
Saliva		
	1. Starch (polysaccharide)	
Gastric Juice		
		2. Partially digested proteins
Pancreatic Juice		
		3. Peptides and amino acids
	4. Fats emulsified by bile	
	5. Starch	
Intestinal Enzymes		
	6. Peptides	
7. Sucrase		
	8. Lactose (milk sugar)	
		9. Glucose

Unscramble the Words

87. Bolus
88. Chyme
89. Papilla
90. Peritoneum
91. Lace apron

Applying What You Know

92. Ulcer
93. Pylorospasm
94. Basal metabolic rate or protein-bound iodine to determine thyroid function

95. WORD FIND

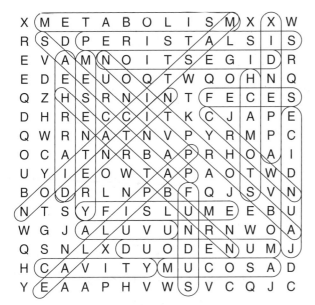

Crossword

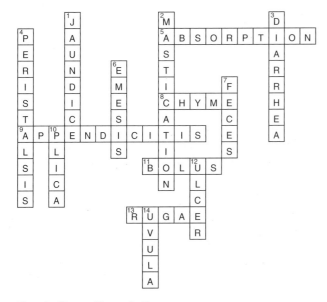

Check Your Knowledge

Multiple Choice

1. a, p. 368
2. c, p. 369
3. a, p. 368
4. b, p. 372
5. b, p. 373
6. b, p. 373
7. b, p. 375
8. c, p. 374
9. c, p. 376
10. a, p. 380

Fill in the Blanks

11. Ileocecal valve, p. 380
12. Sigmoid colon, p. 381
13. Cecum, p. 382
14. Mesentery, p. 383
15. Mechanical digestion, p. 383
16. Monosaccharides, p. 384
17. Amino acids, p. 385
18. Fatty acids, glycerol, p. 385
19. Absorption, p. 385
20. Maltase, sucrase, lactase, p. 385

Digestive Organs

1. Parotid gland
2. Submandibular gland
3. Pharynx
4. Esophagus
5. Diaphragm
6. Transverse colon
7. Hepatic flexure
8. Ascending colon
9. Ileum
10. Cecum
11. Vermiform appendix
12. Rectum
13. Tongue
14. Sublingual gland
15. Larynx
16. Trachea
17. Liver
18. Stomach
19. Spleen
20. Splenic flexure
21. Descending colon
22. Sigmoid colon
23. Anal canal
24. Pancreas
25. Duodenum
26. Gallbladder
27. Cystic duct
28. Common hepatic duct
29. Spleen

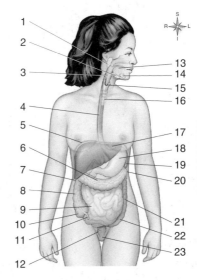

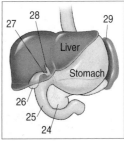

Tooth

1. Cusp
2. Enamel
3. Dentin
4. Pulp cavity with nerves and vessels
5. Gingiva
6. Root canal
7. Peridontal membrane
8. Cementum
9. Bone
10. Root
11. Neck
12. Crown

Stomach

1. Gastroesophageal sphincter
2. Esophagus
3. Gastroesophageal opening
4. Lesser curvature
5. Pylorus
6. Pyloric sphincter
7. Duodenum
8. Rugae
9. Greater curvature
10. Submucosa
11. Mucosa
12. Oblique muscle layer
13. Circular muscle layer
14. Longitudinal muscle layer
15. Serosa
16. Body
17. Fundus

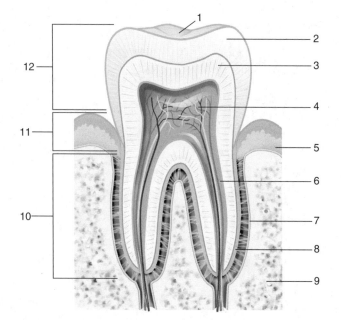

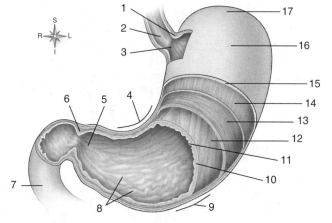

Salivary Glands

1. Parotid gland
2. Parotid duct
3. Submandibular gland
4. Submandibular duct
5. Sublingual gland

Gallbladder and Bile Ducts

1. Corpus (body) of gallbladder
2. Neck of gallbladder
3. Cystic duct
4. Liver
5. Minor duodenal papilla
6. Major duodenal papilla
7. Duodenum
8. Sphincter muscles
9. Superior mesenteric artery and vein
10. Pancreatic duct
11. Pancreas
12. Common bile duct
13. Common hepatic duct
14. Right and left hepatic ducts

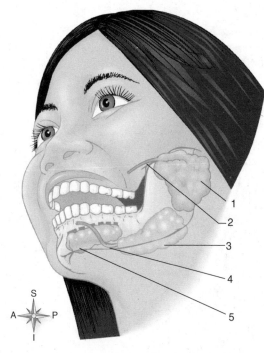

Small Intestine

1. Mesentery
2. Serosa
3. Longitudinal muscle
4. Circular muscle
5. Muscularis
6. Submucosa
7. Plica (fold)
8. Lymph nodule
9. Mucosa
10. Segment of jejunum
11. Microvilli
12. Epithelial cell
13. Single villus
14. Mucosa
15. Microvilli
16. Submucosa
17. Lacteal (lymph capillary)
18. Artery and vein

Large Intestine

1. Aorta
2. Splenic vein
3. Superior mesenteric artery
4. Splenic (left colic) flexure
5. Inferior mesenteric artery and vein
6. Descending colon
7. Sigmoid colon
8. Rectum
9. Mesentery
10. Ileum
11. Vermiform appendix
12. Cecum
13. Ileocecal valve
14. Ascending colon
15. Hepatic (right colic) flexure
16. Transverse colon
17. Inferior vena cava
18. Portal vein

Magnification of jejunal mucosal wall

Two cells of the villus epithelium showing brush border (microvilli)

Mucosal villi

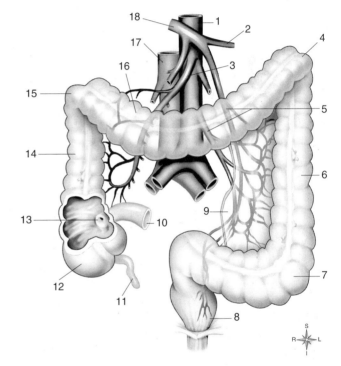

CHAPTER 17
NUTRITION AND METABOLISM

Fill in the Blanks

1. Bile, p. 396
2. Prothrombin, p. 396
3. Fibrinogen, p. 396
4. Iron, p. 397
5. Hepatic portal vein, p. 397

Matching

6. b, p. 399
7. a, p. 397
8. c, p. 400
9. d, p. 400
10. e, p. 401
11. a, p. 397
12. e, p. 401
13. a, p. 397

Select the One That Does Not Belong

14. Bile (the others refer to carbohydrate metabolism)
15. Amino acids (the others refer to fat metabolism)
16. M (the others refer to vitamins)
17. Iron (the others refer to protein metabolism)
18. Insulin (the others tend to increase blood glucose)
19. Folic acid (the others are minerals)
20. Ascorbic acid (the others refer to the B-complex vitamins)

Circle the Correct Answer

21. c, p. 401
22. a, p. 403
23. c, p. 403
24. b, p. 403
25. b, p. 403
26. a, p. 403
27. c, p. 403
28. d, p. 403
29. a, p. 398

Unscramble the Words

30. Liver
31. Catabolism
32. Amino
33. Pyruvic
34. Evaporation

Applying What You Know

35. Weight loss; anorexia nervosa
36. Iron; meat, eggs, vegetables, and legumes
37. She was carbohydrate loading or glycogen loading, which allows the muscles to sustain aerobic exercise for up to 50% longer than usual.

38. WORD FIND

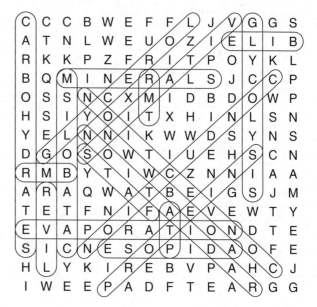

Crossword

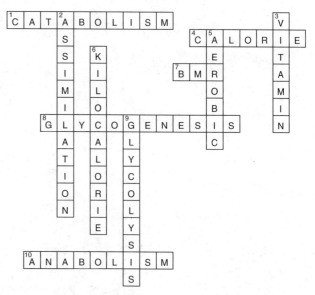

Check Your Knowledge

Multiple Choice

1. b, p. 395
2. a, p. 397
3. c, p. 397
4. c, p. 399
5. b, p. 399
6. b, p. 397
7. a, p. 400
8. a, p. 402
9. b, p. 403
10. d, p. 396

Fill in the Blanks

11. Carbohydrates, p. 397
12. Glycolysis, p. 397
13. Citric acid cycle, p. 398
14. Iodine, p. 402
15. Basal metabolic rate, p. 401
16. Total metabolic rate, p. 403
17. Hypothalamus, p. 403
18. Catabolism, p. 396
19. Anabolism, p. 396
20. A, D, E, K, p. 400

CHAPTER 18
URINARY SYSTEM

Multiple Choice

1. e, p. 411
2. c, p. 411
3. e, p. 411
4. c, p. 413
5. e, p. 415
6. c, p. 415
7. b, p. 415
8. e, p. 415
9. c, p. 416
10. c, p. 417
11. b, p. 418 (review Chapter 11)
12. d, p. 418

Matching

13. g, p. 411
14. i, p. 423
15. h, p. 409
16. b, p. 411
17. k, p. 411
18. f, p. 411
19. j, p. 411
20. d, p. 411
21. l, p. 411
22. c, p. 411
23. m, p. 414
24. a, p. 411

Indicate Which Organ Is Identified

25. b, p. 420
26. c, p. 420
27. a, p. 419
28. b, p. 420
29. c, p. 420
30. c, p. 420
31. a, p. 419
32. c, p. 420
33. b, p. 420
34. a, p. 419
35. b, p. 420

Fill in the Blanks

36. Renal colic, p. 420
37. Mucous membrane, p. 419
38. Renal calculi, p. 419
39. Ultrasound, p. 419
40. Reduced, p. 418
41. Renal pelvis, p. 419
42. Semen, p. 421
43. Urinary meatus, p. 418

Fill in the Blanks

44. Micturition, p. 421
45. Urination, p. 421
46. Voiding, p. 421
47. Internal urethral, p. 421
48. Exit, p. 421
49. Striated, p. 421
50. Voluntary, p. 421
51. Emptying reflex, p. 421
52. Urethra, p. 421
53. Retention, p. 421
54. Suppression, p. 421
55. Stress incontinence, p. 421
56. Routine, p. 423
57. Microscopic, p. 423
58. Disease, p. 423

Unscramble the Words

56. Calyx
57. Voiding
58. Papilla
59. Glomerulus
60. Pyramids

Applying What You Know

61. Polyuria
62. Residual urine is often the cause of repeated cystitis.
63. A high percentage of catheterized patients develop an infection (cystitis), often due to poor aseptic technique when inserting the catheter.
64. WORD FIND

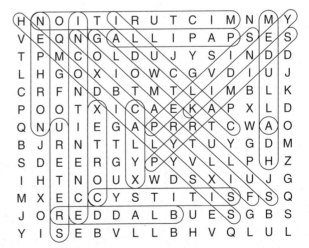

Crossword

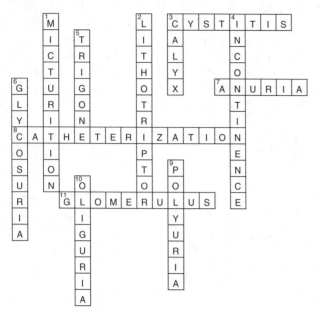

Urinary System

1. Urinary bladder
2. Ureter
3. Right kidney
4. Twelfth rib
5. Liver
6. Adrenal gland
7. Spleen
8. Renal artery
9. Renal vein
10. Left kidney
11. Abdominal aorta
12. Inferior vena cava
13. Common iliac artery and vein
14. Urethra

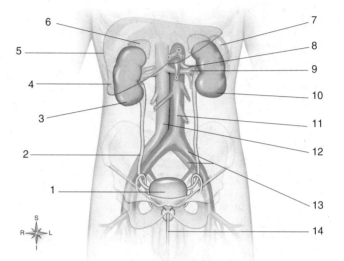

Check Your Knowledge

Multiple Choice

1. d, p. 410
2. b, p. 411
3. d, p. 413
4. a, p. 415
5. c, p. 417
6. c, p. 419
7. b, p. 418
8. c, p. 418
9. b, p. 420
10. a, p. 415

Matching

11. e, p. 409
12. c, p. 411
13. f, p. 411
14. d, p. 414
15. j, p. 417
16. h, p. 414
17. a, p. 420
18. g, p. 421
19. i, p. 411
20. b, p. 411

Kidney

1. Interlobular arteries
2. Renal column
3. Renal sinus
4. Hilum
5. Renal pelvis
6. Renal papilla of pyramid
7. Ureter
8. Medulla
9. Medullary pyramid
10. Major calyces
11. Minor calyces
12. Cortex
13. Capsule (fibrous)

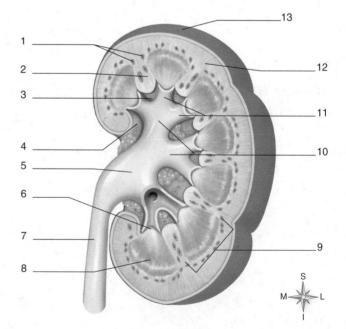

Nephron

1. Proximal convoluted tubule
2. Collecting duct
3. Descending limb of Henle loop
4. Ascending limb of Henle loop
5. Descending limb of Henle loop
6. Artery and vein
7. Distal convoluted tubule
8. Peritubular capillaries
9. Afferent arteriole
10. Juxtaglomerular (JG) apparatus
11. Efferent arteriole
12. Glomerulus
13. Bowman capsule
14. Renal corpuscle

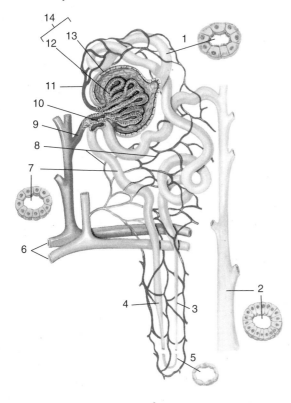

CHAPTER 19
FLUID AND ELECTROLYTE BALANCE

Circle the Correct Answer

1. Inside, p. 431
2. Extracellular, p. 431
3. Extracellular, p. 431
4. Lower, p. 430
5. More, p. 430
6. Decline, p. 430
7. Less, p. 430
8. Decreases, p. 430
9. 55%, p. 430
10. Fluid balance, p. 429

Multiple Choice

11. a, p. 435
12. d, p. 435
13. a, p. 433
14. c, p. 432
15. e, p. 432
16. d, p. 433
17. d, p. 432
18. b, p. 433
19. d, p. 438
20. e, p. 437
21. b, p. 434
22. b, p. 434
23. b, p. 434
24. e, p. 436

True or False

25. Catabolism, not anabolism, p. 432
26. T
27. T
28. Nonelectrolyte, not electrolyte, p. 435
29. Hypervolemia, not hypovolemia, p. 433
30. 2,400 mL, not 1,200 mL, p. 432
31. T
32. 1,000-1,300 mEq, not 500 mL, p. 436

Fill in the Blanks

33. Dehydration, p. 434
34. Decreases, p. 434
35. Decrease, p. 434
36. Overhydration, p. 434
37. Intravenous fluids, p. 435
38. Heart, p. 435

Fill in the Blanks

39. Water, p. 437
40. Hyperkalemia, p. 437
41. Calcium, p. 438
42. Hypercalcemia, p. 438

Unscramble the Words

43. Edema
44. Fluid
45. Ion
46. Intravenous
47. Volume

Applying What You Know

48. Mrs. Titus could not accurately measure water intake created by foods or catabolism, nor could she measure output created by lungs, skin, or the intestines.
49. A careful record of fluid intake and output should be maintained, and the patient should be monitored for signs and symptoms of electrolyte and water imbalance.

50. WORD FIND

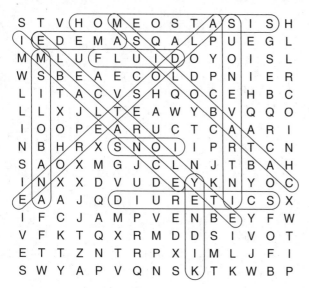

Crossword

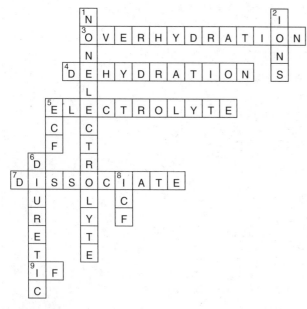

Check Your Knowledge

Multiple Choice

1. a, p. 430
2. d, pp. 432-434
3. d, p. 432
4. c, p. 432
5. a, p. 434
6. b, p. 436
7. d, p. 433
8. a, p. 433
9. a, p. 431
10. d, p. 432

Matching

11. e, p. 431
12. b, p. 431
13. a, p. 435
14. j, p. 435
15. d, p. 438

16. c, p. 429
17. f, p. 436
18. g, p. 434
19. h, p. 435
20. o, p. 433
21. i, p. 434
22. l, p. 433
23. m, p. 435
24. n, p. 436
25. k, p. 435

CHAPTER 20
ACID-BASE BALANCE

Choose the Correct Term

1. b, p. 445
2. a, p. 445
3. a, p. 446
4. b, p. 446
5. b, p. 446
6. b, p. 446
7. a, p. 446
8. a, p. 446
9. b, p. 446
10. b, p. 446

Multiple Choice

11. e, p. 447
12. e, p. 447
13. a, p. 447
14. e, p. 449
15. c, p. 449
16. d, p. 449
17. c, p. 449
18. b, p. 450
19. d, p. 450
20. e, p. 447

True or False

21. Acidosis, not alkalosis, p. 450
22. Buffer, not heart, p. 447
23. Buffer pairs, not duobuffers, p. 447
24. T
25. T
26. Alkalosis, not acidosis, p. 450
27. Kidneys, not lungs, p. 450
28. T
29. Kidneys, not lungs, p. 450
30. Lungs, not kidneys, p. 449

Matching

31. e, p. 452
32. g, p. 451
33. f, p. 452
34. a, p. 451
35. i, p. 452
36. b, p. 451
37. h, p. 451
38. c, p. 451
39. d, p. 451
40. j, p. 451

Unscramble the Words

41. Fluids
42. Bicarbonate
43. Base
44. Fixed
45. Hydrogen
46. Buffer

Applying What You Know

47. Normal saline contains chloride ions, which replace bicarbonate ions and thus relieve the bicarbonate excess that occurs during severe vomiting.
48. Most citrus fruits, although acid-tasting, are fully oxidized during metabolism and have little effect on acid-base balance. Cranberry juice is one of the few exceptions.
49. Milk of Magnesia. It is a base. Milk is slightly acidic (see chart, p. 446).
50. WORD FIND

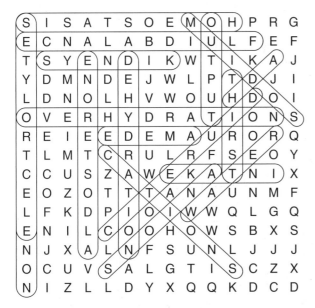

Crossword

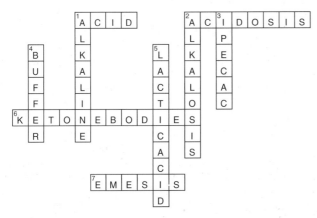

Check Your Knowledge

Multiple Choice

1. a, p. 445
2. c, p. 446
3. a, p. 447
4. d, p. 448

5. a, p. 452
6. d, p. 447
7. d, p. 451
8. d, p. 451
9. d, p. 450
10. d, p. 447

Matching

11. g, p. 446
12. c, p. 446
13. i, p. 450
14. e, p. 448
15. f, p. 447
16. a, p. 451
17. b, p. 447
18. d, p. 450
19. j, p. 451
20. h, p. 451

CHAPTER 21 REPRODUCTIVE SYSTEM

Matching

Group A

1. d, p. 460
2. c, p. 460
3. e, p. 460
4. b, p. 460
5. a, p. 460

Group B

6. c, p. 460
7. a, p. 460
8. d, p. 459
9. b, p. 460
10. e, p. 460

Multiple Choice

11. b, p. 461
12. c, p. 462
13. a, p. 462
14. d, p. 464
15. e, p. 463
16. d, p. 462
17. c, p. 463
18. c, p. 462
19. a, p. 463
20. b, p. 464

Fill in the Blanks

21. Testes, p. 460
22. Spermatozoa or sperm, p. 462
23. Ovum, p. 460
24. Testosterone, p. 462
25. Interstitial cells, p. 462
26. Masculinizing, p. 463
27. Anabolic, p. 463

Choose the Correct Term

28. b, p. 465
29. h, p. 465
30. g, p. 465
31. a, p. 464
32. f, p. 465
33. c, p. 465
34. i, p. 465
35. e, p. 465
36. d, p. 466
37. j, p. 466

Matching

38. d, p. 466
39. c, p. 467
40. b, p. 471
41. a, p. 467
42. e, p. 466

Select the Correct Term

43. a, p. 472
44. b, p. 471
45. a, p. 470
46. b, p. 466
47. a, p. 472
48. a, p. 473
49. a, p. 472
50. b, p. 467

Fill in the Blanks

51. Gonads, p. 467
52. Oogenesis, p. 468
53. Meiosis, p. 462
54. One-half or 23, p. 462
55. Fertilization, p. 468
56. 46, p. 468
57. Estrogen, p. 468
58. Progesterone, p. 468
59. Secondary sexual characteristics, p. 468
60. Menstrual cycle, p. 468
61. Puberty, p. 468

Select the Correct Term

62. a, p. 470
63. b, p. 471
64. c, p. 471
65. b, p. 471
66. a, p. 466; c, p. 471
67. b, p. 466
68. a, p. 466
69. a, p. 470
70. c, p. 471
71. b, p. 471

Matching
Group A

72. d, p. 471
73. e, p. 471
74. b, p. 471
75. c, p. 471
76. a, p. 471

Group B

77. e, p. 472
78. a, p. 473
79. d, p. 473
80. b, p. 473
81. c, p. 473

True or False

82. "Menarche," not "climacteric," p. 473
83. One ovum, not several, p. 475
84. 14, not 28, p. 475
85. Menstrual flow, not ovulation, p. 474
86. T, p. 475
87. Anterior, not posterior, p. 475

Matching

88. b, p. 475
89. a, p. 475
90. b, p. 475
91. b, p. 475
92. a, p. 475

Unscramble the Words

93. Vulva
94. Testes
95. Menses
96. Fimbriae
97. Prepuce
98. Vestibule

Applying What You Know

99. Yes. The testes not only are essential organs of reproduction but are also responsible for the "masculinizing" hormone. Without this hormone, Mr. Belinki will have no desire to reproduce.
100. Sterile. The sperm count may be too low to reproduce but the remaining testicle will produce enough masculinizing hormone to prevent impotence.
101. The uterine tubes are not attached to the ovaries, and infections can exit at this area and enter the abdominal cavity.
102. Yes. Yes. Without the hormones from the ovaries to initiate the menstrual cycle, Mrs. Harlan will no longer have a menstrual cycle and can be considered to be in menopause (cessation of menstrual cycle).
103. No. Christie will still have her ovaries, which are the source of her hormones. She will not experience menopause due to this procedure.

Female Pelvis

1. Uterine (fallopian) tube
2. Ovary
3. Body of uterus
4. Fundus of uterus
5. Urinary bladder
6. Pubic symphysis
7. Urethra
8. Clitoris
9. Vagina
10. Labium minus
11. Labium majus
12. Rectum
13. Cervix
14. Ureter

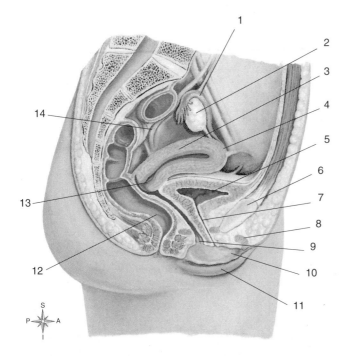

Uterus and Adjacent Structures

1. Fundus
2. Body of uterus
3. Cervix
4. Vagina
5. Cervical canal
6. Perimetrium
7. Myometrium
8. Endometrium
9. Ovary
10. Fimbriae
11. Uterine (fallopian) tube

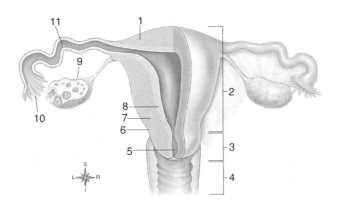

CHAPTER 22
GROWTH, DEVELOPMENT, AND AGING

Fill in the Blanks

1. Conception, p. 486
2. Birth, p. 486
3. Embryology, p. 486
4. Oviduct, fallopian tube, or uterine tube, p. 486
5. Zygote, p. 486
6. Morula, p. 486
7. Blastocyst, p. 486
8. Amniotic cavity, p. 487
9. Chorion, p. 487
10. Placenta, p. 487

Matching

11. g, p. 486
12. f, p. 489
13. c, p. 494
14. b, p. 488
15. a, p. 486
16. h, p. 490
17. e, p. 493
18. d, p. 489
19. i, p. 488
20. j, p. 494

Multiple Choice

21. e, p. 493
22. e, p. 495
23. e, p. 495
24. a, p. 495
25. b, p. 495
26. c, p. 495
27. b, p. 495
28. d, p. 495
29. e, p. 495
30. d, p. 496
31. a, p. 496
32. c, p. 496
33. c, p. 496
34. c, p. 496
35. e, p. 496

Matching

36. f, p. 493
37. a, p. 495
38. c, p. 496
39. h, p. 495
40. d, p. 496
41. b, p. 495
42. e, p. 496
43. g, p. 495
44. i, p. 496

Fill in the Blanks

45. Lipping, p. 497
46. Osteoarthritis, p. 497
47. Nephron, p. 498
48. Barrel chest, p. 498

49. Atherosclerosis, p. 497
50. Arteriosclerosis, p. 497
51. Hypertension, p. 498
52. Presbyopia, p. 497
53. Cataract, p. 497
54. Glaucoma, p. 497

Unscramble the Words

55. Infancy
56. Postnatal
57. Organogenesis
58. Zygote
59. Childhood
60. Fertilization

Applying What You Know

61. Normal
62. Only about 40% of the taste buds present at age 30 remain at age 75.
63. A significant loss of hair cells in the organ of Corti causes a serious decline in ability to hear certain frequencies.
64. WORD FIND

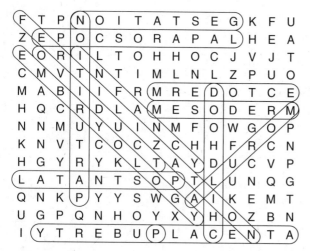

Crossword

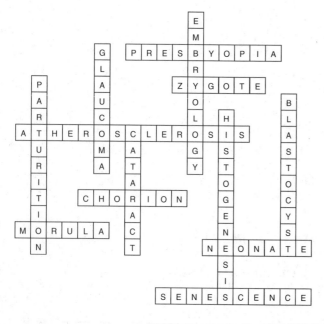

Check Your Knowledge

Multiple Choice

1. c, p. 485
2. d, p. 486
3. d, p. 487
4. a, p. 486
5. d, p. 488
6. d, p. 489
7. c, p. 490
8. a, p. 488
9. c, p. 495
10. b, p. 496

Matching

11. e, p. 490
12. g, p. 486
13. c, p. 488
14. i, p. 496
15. h, p. 490
16. d, p. 493
17. j, p. 497
18. f, p. 497
19. a, p. 496
20. b, p. 495

Fertilization and Implantation

1. Ovary
2. Developing follicles
3. Corpus luteum
4. Fimbriae
5. Discharged ovum
6. Spermatozoa
7. First mitosis
8. Uterine (fallopian) tube
9. Divided zygote
10. Morula
11. Blastocyst
12. Implantation

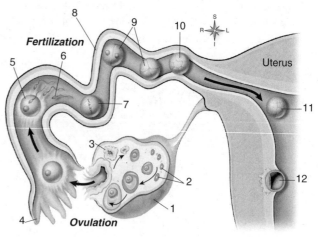